MENTAL
HEALTH
FIRST AID

A practical guide for workplaces, schools, families, friends, carers and everyone needing support with their mental health.

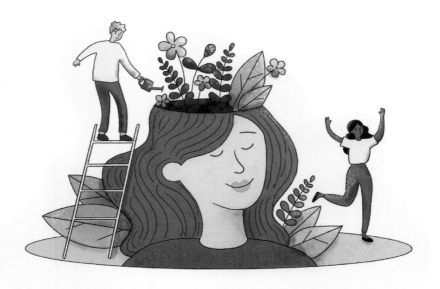

Published by First Aid for Life

Mental Health First Aid has been written by Emma Hammett, qualified nurse, first aid trainer and founder of First Aid for Life and onlinefirstaid.com in conjunction with other medical, first aid, health and emergency services professionals and with special thanks for specific input from Clinicians at Maudsley Learning.

The contents are based on best practice at the time of publication and will be reviewed and updated with new editions.

Disclaimer: the author has made every effort to ensure the accuracy of the information contained within this book and whilst the book offers guidance it does not replace medical help. The author does not accept any liability or responsibility for any inaccuracies or for any mistreatment or misdiagnosis of any person or animal, however caused. If you suspect illness or injury, you should always seek immediate professional medical advice.

MENTAL HEALTH FIRST AID

A practical guide to supporting good mental health – for workplaces, schools, friends, families, carers and everyone wanting to learn more about optimising their mental health and where to get help if struggling.

Introduction

It is estimated that around 1 in 4 people in the UK will experience a mental health condition at some point in their lives. For many, work is a major source of stress that can be detrimental to their mental health. 1 in 6 employees suffer from common mental health problems in the workplace. When businesses proactively support people with their mental health, it can transform the workplace into a more positive and productive working environment.

We know that many mental health conditions develop in childhood and adolescence:

- 20% of adolescents are likely to experience a mental health problem in any given year.

- 50% of mental health problems are established by age 14 and 75% by the age of 24.

- Many children as young as 9 are regularly self-harming.

Therefore, it is critical that schools, colleges, and universities are equipped with the skills to help their pupils (and staff) with their mental wellbeing.

Unfortunately, despite recent campaigns and advances, there still remains a level of stigma and fear of discrimination around mental health conditions. Employees may feel that mental health conditions will not be greeted with the same compassionate approach as physical illness. This should not be the case and the purpose of this course is to demystify mental health conditions and empower workplaces, friends, teachers and family members to provide the support and signposting desperately needed by those struggling with their mental well-being.

The HSE have embraced the idea of mental health in the workplace and issued the following guidance 'First aid needs assessment' for businesses.

They strongly advise that your first aid needs assessment should now include mental health first aid.

There has also been a major drive to raise the profile of mental health awareness in primary and secondary schools and equip more support staff and teachers with the skills to recognise and help appropriately and promptly if a child or young person appears to be struggling with their mental wellbeing.

Most people will struggle to cope at some point in their lives. Therefore, it is critical to equip people with skills to give them the courage to appropriately reach out to someone in need. This caring approach will demonstrate that they are valued, help them access the support they need and could give them a lifeline to restore their mental wellbeing.

The information within this book will teach you how to recognise warning signs of mental ill health and help you develop the skills and confidence to approach and support someone, whilst keeping yourself safe.

We cover how to spot specific warning signs that someone could be struggling with a mental health condition and how to initiate a supportive conversation. We introduce an action plan to help and offer guidance as to when and how to encourage someone to seek appropriate professional help. In addition, we explore other ways to reduce stress and boost mental health and identify the multitude of self-help and support options available.

The scope of this information is not to learn how to diagnose or treat mental health conditions as this should only be done by appropriately trained healthcare professionals. However, you will be guided in identifying signs that someone might be struggling and we will equip you with a methodology to appropriately support them and a directory of charities, organisations and online forums where you can signpost them for help.

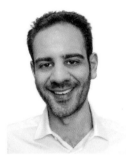

"Mental Health First Aid is a superb manual. The CARES approach used by First Aid for Life can be applied to any situation where you encounter someone in distress, whether in public, your workplace, or personal life. This simple intervention may be profound and lifesaving".

Dr Greg Shields, Consultant Liaison Psychiatrist, South London and Maudsley NHS Foundation Trust and Maudsley Learning

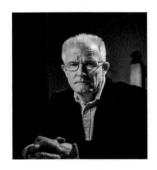

"As the stigma surrounding mental illness continues to recede, we welcome this comprehensive and practical guide to psychological disorder and mental healthcare. A real resource for real people in the real world."

Steve Mallen, Co-Founder, Zero Suicide Alliance

The information in this book is at a level equivalent to Level 1 RQF/ Level 4 SCQF.

Foreword

Many people will experience an episode of mental ill health during their lifetime, ranging from mild depression or anxiety to severe and chronic mental illness. Decades of campaigning by non-government organisations supported by high-profile individuals and mental health professionals, together with significant progress in media portrayal of mental illness, has meant that we now talk about mental ill health more openly and more often. We are now more sensitive to others' psychological distress. The prevalence of abuse on social media and the COVID pandemic are two recent developments that have brought mental illness into focus and heightened the need for us to actively support one another.

Mental health first aid has the same goals as its physical health counterpart: giving ordinary people the basic skills needed to assess and assist when there are concerns that someone is at risk or in crisis. After taking this training you should feel confident to approach someone to help with their wellbeing and welfare, provide reassurance and comfort in the moment, and seek help where and when appropriate. The CARES approach used by First Aid for Life can be applied to any situation in which you encounter someone in distress, whether in public, your workplace, or personal life. This simple intervention may be profound and lifesaving.

Contents

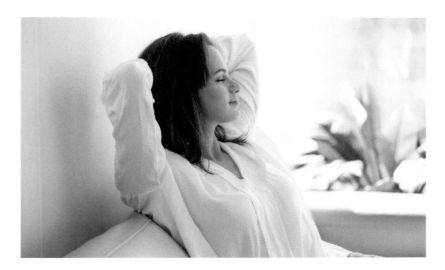

What is Mental Health?

Mental health involves all aspects of our emotional, psychological and social well-being. How our brain is feeling, affects how we think, feel and act. It is also fundamental to our ability to handle stress, relate to others and function on a day to day basis. Mental health encompasses a range of states and can vary from day to day or moment to moment, depending on external and internal elements. The state of someone's mental health can affect all aspects of someone's life:

- A deterioration in mental health is often inextricably linked with a deterioration in physical health.

- Poor mental health makes it harder for people to function at their best at work.

- As parents or spouses (it can have a profound effect on intimate relationships and the ability to support one another)

- Whilst studying, if still in education.

- Often medication prescribed for mental health conditions can affect someone's ability to operate machinery safely at work, or to drive.

Mental illness is treatable with a multitude of different therapies that might involve talking, medication, or lifestyle changes. There are also a huge range of supportive organisations and support groups for specific conditions.

The following definition of mental health helps us appreciate how fundamental our mental wellbeing is to how we function as individuals: **"Mental health influences how we think and feel about ourselves and others and how we interpret events. It affects our capacity to learn, to communicate, and to form, sustain and end relationships. It also influences our ability to cope with change, transition and life events: having a baby, moving house, experiencing bereavement."**

Friedli L Mental health improvement concepts and definitions 2004

If the above is a definition of mental health, then conversely mental ill health is where the person is no longer in control of their emotions and may struggle to cope with change, relationships and stress.

The Mental Health Continuum

Mental health conditions are described as being on a continuum – like having various grades or shades of well-being. Although there are extremes of health and illness, generally physical and mental health conditions exist on a spectrum. Mental and physical health conditions can be acute and chronic. For example, just as with a chronic health condition such as Asthma; chronic mental health conditions can be well managed, and people continue to live life to the full.

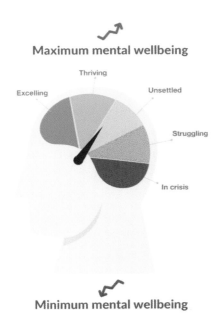

Maximum mental wellbeing

Thriving

Excelling   Unsettled

Struggling

In crisis

Minimum mental wellbeing

Some people only experience one episode of mental illness in their entire life; some have multiple episodes of illness with gaps of wellness in-between. It is extremely rare to have ongoing mental health issues that can't be managed or improved at all. As with physical illness, generally the sooner someone identifies there is a problem and seeks appropriate help, the better the prognosis.

It is perfectly normal to feel down, stressed or frightened. Most of the time those feelings pass, but occasionally they develop into a mental health problem such as anxiety or depression; these can be hard to cope with and may impact on our daily lives. For some people, mental health problems become complex, and require support and treatment for life. Factors like poverty, genetics, childhood trauma, abuse, discrimination, or ongoing physical illness have been shown to make mental health problems more likely, but anyone can experience a mental health issue.Sadly, over 6,000 people a year die by suicide in the UK

Our mental health is often impacted by our physical health and vice versa. Sometimes increasing amounts of stress can lead us to struggle to cope. There is a huge range of mental ill health and mental health issues – many are not diagnosable and are part of a normal continuum. The methods and approaches discussed within this book are applicable to most situations involving people trying to maintain or attain good mental health.

Anyone can experience a form of mental illness, but some factors make it more likely that someone could be affected:

- An increase in stress or long-term stress

- Abuse, trauma, neglect or feeling unloved

- Unemployment or losing your job

- Experiencing a long-term physical health problem or life-changing injury

- Social isolation or loneliness

- Poverty, money struggles or homelessness

- Being a home carer

- Drug or alcohol abuse

- Domestic violence

- Post traumatic experience – particularly prevalent in some jobs, such as the Military, paramedics and other emergency services

- Bereavement

How common are mental health issues?

Research has shown that one in four people will experience some form of mental health issue during the course of a year. One of the largest surveys in England conducted in 2016 suggested that one in six people experience the symptoms of a mental health problem in any given week.

(McManus, S., Bebbington, P., Jenkins, R., & Brugha, T. (Eds.) (2016). Mental health and wellbeing in England: Adult Psychiatric Morbidity Survey 2014)

It is thought that three quarters of all mental health problems have become established by the age of 24. But frighteningly half of all mental health problems become apparent by the age of 14.

1 in 10 children aged 5-16 have a diagnosable mental health condition (but only a fraction of these will have been diagnosed or offered help).

In the developed world, anxiety is the most common mental illness, followed by mood disorders such as depression and then issues resulting from substance misuse – including alcohol and drugs.

Generally, it is women who experience more anxiety issues and men more substance misuse. However, it is not unusual for the disorders to occur in combination (often termed dual diagnosis, co-morbidity or co-occurrence), such as situations where someone who is depressed misuses alcohol, or someone with an anxiety disorder, also feels depressed.

Mental Health and children and young people

Poor mental health among children and young people rose between 2004 & 2016: from 1 in 10 to 1 in 8 (and in 2020 to 1 in 6)

Childhood mental health problems are extremely common, can be very persistent and unfortunately it is not as easy as it should be to get the necessary help.

We have a specific Mental Health First Aid course focussing on helping children and young people.

There is also a chapter in this book for friends, family, parents, carers and school staff specifically written to help you start difficult conversations and support the young person you care about to get the help they need.

Laws protecting our health, mental health and wellbeing

There is legislation designed to protect people and help care for their mental and physical well-being:

National Institute for Health and Care Excellence (NICE) have evidence-based guidance and quality standards for treatment and management of mental health conditions.

Health and Safety at Work Act 1974 – legislation that requires employers to care for the health, safety and welfare of their employees at work.

Mental Health Act 1983 – covers assessment, treatment and rights of people with mental health disorders. The Act also governs when someone can be 'sectioned' for their own safety or those of others.

The Care Act 2014 The Care Act helps to improve people's independence and wellbeing. It makes clear that local authorities must provide or arrange services that help prevent people developing needs for care and support or delay people deteriorating such that they would need ongoing care and support. https://www.gov. uk/government/publications/care-act-2014-part-1-factsheets/ care-act-factsheets

The law and consent

Act, if they believe their refusal to accept treatment might result in death or serious injury.

Your responsibility

There is no legal requirement in the UK to stop and help strangers in the street.

Workplace responsibility

However, there are UK laws with regards to looking after your own and each other's health and safety whilst in the workplace.

Professional responsibility

Certain professions such as doctors and nurses have a legal duty of care to help in emergency situations.

Reluctance to help

People are often reluctant to help because of concerns they could be sued if they do something wrong. However, no-one in the UK has been successfully sued for trying to 'do the right thing' as long as they didn't step outside of their scope of practice i.e. – no tracheostomy or open heart surgery at the roadside unless you are working as a paramedic and appropriately trained to do it.

A good rule of thumb is to 'stick to the basics'.

Protection against being sued

SOCIAL ACTION, RESPONSIBILITY AND HEROISM BILL (SARAH or the Good Samaritan Act) is there to protect people from being sued if they are providing help and acting with good intent.

In Summary

If someone is unconscious – they need your help and should not pose any threat to your safety. You have presumed consent to go ahead and help within the realms of your knowledge and training.

If someone is conscious but you feel uncomfortable helping them (or they do not want your help), contact the emergency services and watch discretely from a safe distance.

Do trust your instincts though and remain alert and wary, as all may not be as it seems!

Stigma

Unfortunately, there is considerable misinformation concerning mental health and many people are ill-informed and unfoundedly scared of people with a diagnosis of having a mental illness. Many derogatory terms are used to describe people in crisis, and this results in people being reticent about seeking help. Many people mistakenly believe that mental illness is untreatable and will result in someone being admitted to some form of an institution. There is also an unfounded societal belief that people diagnosed with a mental health disorder are out of control, violent and dangerous.

Sadly, these societal beliefs often result in people delaying getting the help they so desperately need. They are worried about the stigma of being diagnosed and 'labelled' as suffering from a mental illness. Often, they try to hide their condition from friends, family and employers. This can sometimes result in them developing a form of self-stigmatisation and isolation.

Family, friends, work and support groups can in fact be a lifeline, once someone has taken the important step of talking about how they are feeling and seeking further help.

Attitudes have begun to change with many celebrities (including Royalty) sharing their own mental health stories and campaigning to encourage people to open up about mental health issues. Things are changing and there is consequently more help available.

However, many people do remain worried about seeking help and frightened as to how family, friends, schools and employers may react.

This is why it is so important that more people read books such as this, to further understand the nature of mental health issues. To appreciate that people can recover from mental illness, but need help and encouragement to seek the necessary professional support.

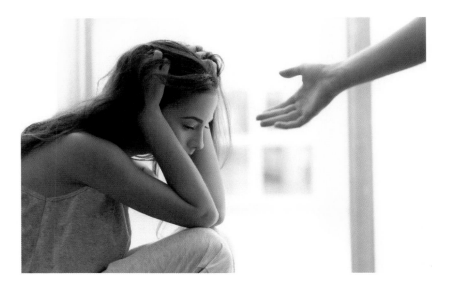

The first aid approach to mental health

We are all aware of the importance of first aid: giving immediate help to someone following an injury or illness.

The aim of first aid is to:

- Preserve life

- Prevent things getting worse

- Promote recovery

- Provide comfort

This is no different when providing first aid for a mental health condition. Understanding how to help someone who is struggling with their mental health or experiencing a mental health issue follows the same principles:

Preserve life – particularly if they are at risk of harming themselves or others

Provide immediate help to prevent the condition worsening

Promote recovery to good mental health

Provide comfort to someone in distress from their mental health condition

First aid is typically provided by a lay person, such as a work colleague or family member and it can be daunting to know the best way to help. That is why people attend first aid courses, to gain the skills and knowledge to be able to help in a medical emergency.

In the same way, it is beneficial to learn about mental health first aid as there are structured ways to approach the situation, which can make it easier to help. Conversely approaching someone the wrong way, could make things more difficult.

We do not attempt to teach people to diagnose possible mental health conditions; however (just as with physical first aid) understanding various conditions is fundamental to offering the right assistance, in the best possible way. It is also essential to signpost people to the most appropriate professional resources in the short and long term.

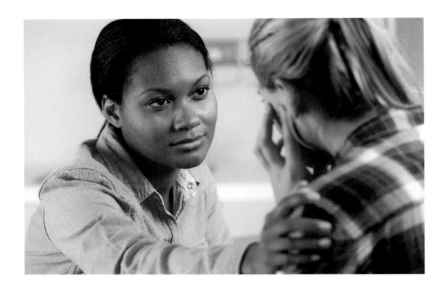

What is a mental health first aider?

The idea behind a mental health first aider is to have someone suitably trained to help. They should be equipped with basic knowledge about mental health conditions, the ability and empathy to spot someone is struggling, and be able to encourage them to seek appropriate help. They should also have access to a wealth of resources to be able to signpost them to the most appropriate help available.

The requirement for a mental health first aider should now be considered as part of all businesses' first aid at work risk assessment. The Health and Safety Executive (HSE) now include the provision of Mental Health First Aid in their First Aid Needs Assessment. https://www.hse.gov.uk/pubns/priced/l74.pdf#page=9

Primary, secondary schools, colleges and universities are also taking serious steps to undertake appropriate training to improve the mental wellbeing of their students (and staff).

A mental health first aider should:

- be an appropriate person to act in a confidential and professional manner to support someone in need of help

- be appropriately trained to be able to recognise signs someone may be struggling with their mental health and be confident approaching them in a non-judgemental way.

- have sufficient up to date knowledge of the most appropriate resources and personnel to signpost the person to, in order to receive the right help.

- have the right knowledge to recognise signs of acute crisis, such as self-harm or risk of suicide and instigate immediate emergency help.

- work in conjunction with management to be able to offer quick solutions to help pre-empt a crisis situation, by being able to adjust workload, reorganise working practices and provide quick, short-term solutions to relieve stress and give the person struggling with their mental health, time to breathe and think clearer.

• work with the organisation and staff to promote awareness of good mental health and consequently reduce stigma for anyone needing help.

• be known by all member of the organisation as the go-to member of the team for these problems – with signage the same way as for a physical first aider.

• actively promote healthy workplace policies for good mental health and be invited to actively participate within meetings discussing changes in working practices, hours, roles…that could increase any aspect of workplace stress and look for ways of supporting staff through these processes.

• Operate in a 100% confidential manner. The only time they may share information without explicit consent is if they are seriously concerned about human safety.

Common treatments and sources of help:

Early intervention when someone is only just showing signs of struggling with their mental health can make a major difference to their recovery.

Prevention programmes and early intervention, such a parenting classes, family support, drug education, resilience programmes in schools, stress management, mental health awareness, have had a positive impact in reducing the numbers of people experiencing mental health crises.

Medication can be prescribed to enhance mood, reduce anxiety, reduce psychotic episodes. However, with all medication there is a risk benefit ratio and it is important to be aware of possible side-effects and ensure the medication is taken appropriately, avoiding possible drug interactions and contra-indications.

Some medication can affect sexual performance, or make your skin more prone to sunburn; they can affect your ability to drive, your mood and energy and ability to safely operate machinery at work.

All these factors need to be carefully considered and discussed before embarking on medication.

Psychological therapies: Talking with a mental health professional 1:1, or in a group session. For some people, these can be incredibly powerful. They are also accessible as apps, skype and zoom consultations, self-help books and courses. They are designed to help people gain self-help coping strategies, insight and find new ways of managing their condition.

There are numerous **complementary therapies** and **lifestyle changes** that can be prescribed by community health professionals or just accessed as self-help. Exercise and changes in diet, both have major roles to play in our mental health.

Support groups can be extremely helpful, MIND have a large online community Side By Side and access to many other support groups from their excellent website.

Rehabilitation programmes help people to re-build confidence and regain skills to be able to live independently.

Family, friends and work-colleagues can play an important role in someone's recovery.

The understanding and support of a **Mental Health First Aider** can be pivotal to the person's ability to cope in the workplace.

Other professionals who can help:

The community health team:

GPs can offer a holistic approach to helping someone with a mental health issue. They can exclude any physical cause, explain how the disease might manifest itself and progress, and prescribe medication and complementary therapies, through social prescribing networks.

Community psychiatric support and **psychologists** can also be helpful in supporting the person's recovery, along with other community support.

Counsellors, psychologists and psychotherapists: have also been proven to help people find new coping mechanisms with their illness. They offer various talking therapies that are specific to different conditions. Sometimes they focus on helping people cope with their conditions and sometimes the focus is more about problem solving, to assist them to solve stressful situations in their lives to cope better. This therapy can be conducted as 1:1 or in groups or families.

Psychiatrists: are medically trained doctors, specialising in treating mental illness. Their focus is usually more medication focussed and they would be more likely to see people with more complex or long-term conditions. Your GP can refer someone to a psychiatrist if they are experiencing more complex illness or are not responding to first line treatment. Although it is possible to access this help privately.

Mental health nurses: specially trained nurses focussing on caring for the mentally ill.

Occupational therapists: Can help re-train people, and make appropriate workplace adjustments to help them return to work.

Care Co-ordinators – or key workers are community based workers who co-ordinate care under the Care Programme Approach CPA and assist a multi-disciplinary team to communicate and work together to help the person cope in the community and workplace.

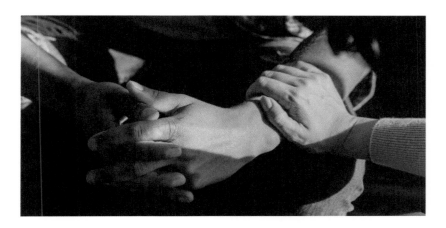

The importance of getting help early:

Just as with physical illness, if people delay getting help with mental health issues, it can delay their recovery.

If someone recognises that someone is struggling with their mental health, approaching them in the right way and prompting them to seek help can lead them to get help quicker.

Sometimes people don't realise they are having problems as they don't have the insight into their condition. People close to them can helpfully facilitate them gaining the help they need.

Signs someone may be struggling with their mental health (remember any of these could also have a physical cause and a visit to their GP is often the most sensible first step):

- Apathy, exhaustion and tiredness for no apparent reason.

- Underperforming at work, for no apparent reason. Maybe losing concentration, slower completing tasks

- Losing interest and a wish to participate in activities that were previously anticipated and enjoyed.

- Loss of appetite or changes in the approach to food – maybe binge-eating or seeking comfort food.

- Increasing anxiety, a panicky feeling in the chest or restlessness.

- Wishing to isolate and hide away.

- Difficulty sleeping.

- Hallucinating or changes in perception meaning you are hearing or seeing things others cannot.

- Self-harming or acting in an uncharacteristically reckless way.

- An increasing reliance on alcohol or recreational drugs.

- Change in sex drive.

The importance of a mental health action plan:

If you believe someone is experiencing symptoms of mental ill health, you should approach the person appropriately and offer help. Getting this right can be difficult and an action plan or more structured method, can make this easier.

For physical first aid, the structure would be DRABC – Check for Danger, check for Response, open the Airway, check for Breathing and Circulation.

For Mental Health First Aid use CARES – a mental health first aid action plan:

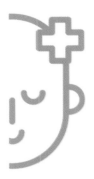

C **Check** to ensure there is no immediate life-threatening crisis. **Calmly** approach, reassure, assess & assist

A **Actively** Listen without judgment

R **Recommend** sources of immediate help – be particularly aware of signs of crisis

E **Encourage** to seek professional help

S **Suggest** possible self-help and other support options for better mental health

Most people will struggle to cope at some point in their lives. This is why it is critical to equip people with skills and courage to appropriately reach out to someone in need. The supportive approach will demonstrate that they are valued, help them access the support they need and could give them the lifeline they need to restore their mental wellbeing.

Everyone copes and reacts in their own way, but there are some general signs that could signal someone might need help:

Signs to look out for

- Feeling restless and agitated

- Feeling angry and aggressive

- Feeling tearful

- Being tired or lacking in energy

- Not wanting to talk to or be with people

- Not wanting to do things they usually enjoy

- Using alcohol or drugs to cope with feelings

- Finding it hard to cope with everyday things

- Not replying to messages or being distant

- Talking about feeling hopeless, helpless or worthless

- Talking about feeling trapped by life circumstances they can't see a way out of, or feeling unable to escape their thoughts

- A change in routine, such as sleeping or eating more or less than normal

- Engaging in risk-taking behaviour, like gambling or violence

You might not always be able to spot these signs and people often try to hide them too.

It can also be useful to identify circumstances that can trigger suicidal thoughts or make it hard for someone to cope.

Stressful life situations that mean someone may need additional support:

- loss, including loss of a friend or a family member through bereavement

- suicide or attempted suicide of family member, friend, or public figure

- relationship or family problems

- housing problems

- financial worries

- job-related stress

- college or study-related pressures

- leaving home, starting a new school, college or job

- bullying, abuse, or neglect

- loneliness and isolation

- challenging current events

- depression

- painful and/or disabling physical illness

- heavy use of or dependency on alcohol or other drugs

Some people appear to cope well with these extreme circumstances. For other people their mental health struggles may appear to occur suddenly with no apparent cause.

The CARES Approach

Check to ensure there is no immediate life-threatening crisis. **C**almly approach, reassure, assess & assist

Actively listen without judgment

Recommend sources of immediate help – be particularly aware of signs of crisis

Encourage to seek professional help

Suggest possible self-help and other support options for better mental health

The Samaritans have some incredibly helpful resources: https://www.samaritans.org/how-we-can-help/if-youre-worried-about-someone-else/how-support-someone-youre-worried-about/

MIND has a page of helpful pointers that may be useful for someone reticent about speaking about a possible mental health issue: seeking help for a mental health problem

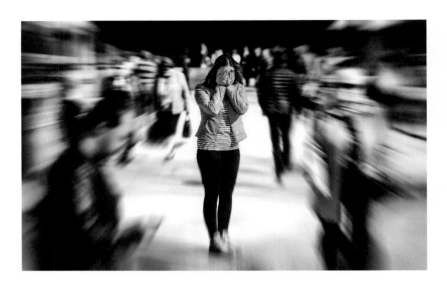

Approaching during a crisis:

An example of a mental health crisis could be if someone is extremely psychotic, or they feel they might attempt suicide or severely harm themselves or someone else. They are demonstrating signs that they are seriously mentally unwell.

If you are approaching someone who you believe may be experiencing a mental health crisis, you may need to move fast to get them appropriate help. If you are concerned that they are an immediate danger to yourself or themselves – and think your approach could escalate this, stay back and observe from a safe distance. Phone 999 and tell them of your concerns. They will send the most appropriate help.

Never put yourself or others at risk of harm.

Possible crises could be the following:

- Fearing that the person may harm themselves – by self-harm, alcohol or drug misuse

- The person is hallucinating or experiencing an extreme psychotic state

- They are extremely distressed and having a serious panic attack

- They are aggressive, disruptive and have lost touch with reality.

Indications that someone may be suicidal:

- Speaking or writing about death, suicide or dying

- Threatening to seriously hurt or kill themselves

- Telling you they would like their life to end

- Increasing use and dependence on drugs or alcohol

- Mood swings and inconsequential or reckless behaviour

- Withdrawing from friends and family

If you think someone is in crisis, MIND has some useful resources to help them cope whilst waiting for help https://www.mind.org.uk/need-urgent-help/what-can-i-do-to-help-myself-cope/getting-through-the-next-few-hours/

Coping exercises and videos https://www.mind.org.uk/need-urgent-help/what-can-i-do-to-help-myself-cope/relaxing-and-calming-exercises/

Help with scary thoughts or hallucinations https://www.mind.org.uk/need-urgent-help/what-can-i-do-to-help-myself-cope/coping-with-scary-thoughts/

Having established that there is no immediate life-threatening emergency. If you do not feel the person is in crisis, but think they could benefit from your help, we suggest you do the following:

1: Calmly approach, assess and assist the person.

Calmly approach them and assess the situation.

Choose a quiet room, where you won't be interrupted, where they will feel relaxed and more able to open up.

Respect their right not to want to discuss things. It could be because they are not ready to talk, it could be because they do not see you as the most appropriate person to open up to, or maybe they don't realise there is a problem, or possibly there has been a miscommunication and you have misread signs.

Carefully choose the best time and place to speak with them

Be sensitive and culturally aware – avoid doing anything that could offend, be misconstrued or could be considered culturally insensitive.

Don't be worried about asking them how they are feeling and how long they have been feeling this way.

2: Actively listen without judgement

This is the first step to someone recognising there may be a problem and that they might need help, is of vital importance. It is critical that they appreciate you are listening in a totally non-judgemental and confidential way and they can speak openly without any worry about prejudice, stigma or implications.

Try not to make assumptions, be patient and non-judgemental.

Think about your body language, where you are sitting and how you can make them feel most at ease.

It is important to ensure the person feels you are listening to them completely and concentrating on what they are saying.

Ensure you are not distracted or interrupted during this important communication.

Set-aside any pre-conceived judgements and ensure you listen to them with a completely open mind.

Use verbal and non-verbal listening and communication skills to ensure that the person knows you are actively listening to them and engaging in what they are saying.

Do not be tempted to interrupt them or to suggest how they may be feeling.

Empathise through gestures and body language.

Accept what the person is saying, even if it doesn't make sense from your perspective.

Try not to jump in and offer solutions

Never give examples of someone else with similar problems as that is seriously breaching confidentiality and will dent their trust and confidence in you too.

Clarify and repeat back what they have told you, so you are both sure you have understood and summarised the situation properly.

3. Recommend sources of immediate help

Once the person has felt they have been listened to and better understood, it may make it easier for the Mental Health First Aider to offer further support and information.

The Mental Health First Aider should make it clear they recognise how the person is feeling and explain how they can help them to regain control of their mental health.

The person may initially need practical help with work or study tasks that feel overwhelming, or there may be something else practical that can be sorted to help ease their stress. Examples might be help with childcare, support with a domestic abuse situation, or supporting them in making an appointment with their GP if the stress is to do with investigating a physical problem – such as a possible tumour.

The Mental Health First Aider should be ready to signpost the person to additional support, if the time is right and the person is not too overwhelmed with their current distress.

It is extremely courageous of them to open up to you and not an easy thing to do. They are likely to feel worried and vulnerable and uncertain as to whether there are any negative implications to the conversation. Reassure them, thank them for confiding and explain, they are not alone – 1 in 4 people experience these feelings and you are here to help.

4. Encourage to seek professional help

Someone with a mental health issue will generally recover faster with appropriate professional help. The Mental Health First Aider should be able to signpost the person to suitable sources of help.

Exploring possible options may enable the Mental Health First Aider to allay fears of possible stigma, or mistaken beliefs about various options.

Helping the person to realise that they are not suffering alone, can be empowering for them. They may not have known about possible options; including counselling, psychological therapy, medication, financial support, help for family members, and specific support groups.

Friend or family member – who knows the person well and is able to help. Maybe a great advocate and support at this time.

Their GP – can offer ongoing holistic support and treatment and refer to appropriate professionals as necessary. They will also be able to rule out medical reasons for the way the person is feeling.

Crisis Line – they may have already been given the Crisis Line number. If so, there will be a trained healthcare professional who should be able to help them.

Samaritans – 116 123 – open 24 hours a day, 365 days a year. With trained operators ready to help.

NHS 111 or 999 if seriously worried that they are a risk to themselves or others.

Reasons to contact the emergency services:

The person is experiencing serious suicidal thoughts or feelings

They are thinking or talking about harming themselves or someone else

Experiencing acute medical symptoms

They have already hurt themselves

You are feeling threatened by their behaviour and our worried that in approaching you could aggravate the situation and put yourself, or them at greater risk.

Please note: It is vital to respect the person's consent. They cannot be forced to seek help or to go to A&E. It is quite common for people to periodically have suicidal thoughts, but never act on them.

5. Suggest possible self-help options for better mental health

Explain other possible self-help strategies

Help them explore specific support groups

Encourage them to discuss how they are feeling with close friends and family

Signpost them to appropriate community and voluntary sector organisations, there are online communities and peer support networks. All there to help. MIND is a superb website to explore together.

Look at proven self-help coping mechanisms

Respect the person's wishes if they prefer to seek culturally-based care.

MIND has some excellent resources to help someone experiencing a mental health issue https://www.mind.org.uk/information-support/helping-someone-else/ and a huge range of specific topics for the person experiencing the mental health issue to access themselves https://www.mind.org.uk/information-support/.

Supporting someone with their mental health and caring for yourself:

Providing help and assistance to someone experiencing a mental health issue can be draining. Ensure you have an appropriate and confidential support network. If you are a mental health first aider in the workplace, your employer should make provision to ensure you receive the support you need to ensure that this additional responsibility does not adversely impact on your well-being.

Try not to get involved personally with the situation you are supporting. Your role is to signpost the person to the most appropriate help.

If you do speak with anyone else about what has happened, ensure you respect the person's privacy, confidentiality and dignity at all times. Do not reveal their identity or share any personal details following your conversation.

The only time it may be appropriate to reveal the person with the mental health issues' identity is when you genuinely feel that the person could be experiencing a crisis and at risk to themselves of others. It would therefore be vital to escalate the situation to get urgent professional help.

Ensure you take time out for yourself to look after your own mental and physical well-being.

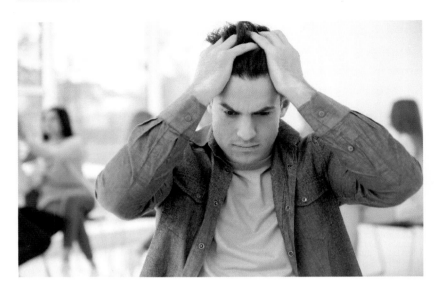

Stress - at home, school or further education and in the workplace

Stress is a reaction to events or experiences in someone's home life, work life or a combination of both. Common mental health problems can have a single cause outside work, for example bereavement, divorce, postnatal depression, a medical condition or a family history of the problem. But people can have these sorts of problems with no obvious causes.

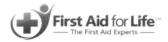
First Aid for Life™
— The First Aid Experts —

Headaches
Raised blood pressure can cause headaches + increase the risk of stroke.

Heartburn
Stress diverts blood away from the gut and reduces the mucosal protection from stomach acid. Therefore any acid remaining in the stomach can lead to discomfort, heartburn and stomach ulcers.

Rapid breathing
An increase in cortisol means you breathe faster.

Risk of heart attack
Stress increases heart rate and increases blood pressure. This increases pressure on your heart.

Fertility problems
Increased stress can interfere with the reproductive system in both men and women, and may make it harder to conceive

Erectile dysfunction
Stress can lead to problems getting and sustaining an erection.

Missed periods
Extreme stress can affect your menstrual cycle and sometimes can cause periods to stop altogether.

Anxiety & depression
Chronic stress can wear you down and also trigger any underlying mental health struggles.

Weakened immune system
Long-term stress can weaken the immune system, leaving you more vulnerable to infections.

High blood sugar
Stress causes your liver to release extra sugar (glucose) into your bloodstream, which raises sugar levels + increases the risk for type 2 diabetes.

High blood pressure
Stress hormones constrict blood vessels, which can raise your blood pressure.

Stomachache
The fight, flight + fright response attacks your digestive system, which can lead to stomachaches, nausea, and other tummy troubles.

Low sex drive
Stress and fatigue can reduce your libido.

Tense muscles
Stress causes muscles to tighten and can lead to aching muscles, including backache and tension headaches.

© www.firstaidforlife.org.uk

43

It is likely that one in four people in the UK will have a mental health problem at some point. Most mental health problems are mild, short term events that are managed with additional support and possibly medication from a family doctor.

Mental health encompasses how we think, feel and behave.

Anxiety and depression are the most common mental health problems. These are often triggered by difficult life events, such as bereavement, having a new baby, a split from a long-term relationship, a stressful home life or medical illness, however they can also be caused by work-related issues.

As outlined above, prolonged stress, whether from home or work, can lead to physical and psychological damage and result in anxiety and depression.

Work-related stress can aggravate an existing mental health problem, making it more difficult to control. Once work-related stress triggers an existing mental health problem, it becomes hard to separate one from the other.

Common mental health problems and stress can exist independently – people can be subject to prolonged stress and physical changes such as high blood pressure, without experiencing anxiety, depression or any other diagnosable mental health problems. They can also develop anxiety and depression without being subject to any stress. It is important to realise when stress and mental health problems are aggravating one another as it may make a difference to the approach taken when a health professional is offering treatment solutions.

Self-help to reduce the impact of stress

19 Proven Ways to Reduce Stress and Anxiety

Prolonged stress is bad for us. It raises our cortisol levels and can manifest itself as a physical and mental health problem. The increase in cortisol levels, leaves us in a continual state of alertness, ready to jump into a fight, flight or fright response. This prolonged rise in cortisol levels is detrimental to our health. It often results in high blood pressure and puts additional strain on the blood vessels in the heart and brain. It has been documented that prolonged stress can lead to structural changes in the brain too

Many people suffer from stress headaches, heartburn, backache; they are unable to sleep and are more prone to infections as stress interferes with their immune system. Stress can increase their blood sugar as it causes your liver to release glucose; it can adversely affect your sexual performance, make you more at risk of a heart attack or stroke and has been shown to be a contributor to mental health problems.

If you are stressed, whether by your job or something more personal, the first step to feeling better is to identify the cause.

The most destructive approach is to turn to something unhealthy to help you cope, such as smoking, drinking or binge-eating comfort food.

Exercise

Stress hormones: Exercise actually lowers your body's stress hormones – such as cortisol. It also helps release endorphins, which are chemicals that boost mood and can act as natural painkillers.

Sleep: Exercise can also improve your sleep quality, which can be adversely affected by stress and anxiety.

Confidence: regular exercise has been shown to contribute to mental wellbeing.

Deep breathing exercises

Cortisol in your bloodstream activates your sympathetic nervous system, signalling the fright, flight or fight response.

In response to this, your heart will beat faster, your breathing quicken and your blood vessels constrict to conserve blood flow to your vital organs.

Controlling your breathing to override this response, will activate your parasympathetic nervous system and help you relax.

The goal of deep breathing is to focus your awareness on your breath, making it slower and deeper. When you breathe in deeply through your nose, your lungs fully expand and your belly rises. There are several types of deep breathing exercises, including diaphragmatic breathing, abdominal breathing, belly breathing and paced respiration.

Understanding how to control your breathing is extremely helpful in combating panic attacks.

Often mindfulness courses and Yoga will incorporate deep breathing exercises.

Take control

Feeling a loss of control is a key contributor to that panicky feeling.

The act of taking control is empowering in its own right and depending on the reason for the stress, may instantly relieve some of the panic

Say no

This is part of taking control. Simplifying the number of things you are doing and who you are trying to please, should help reduce the stress in your life.

Alongside this – delegate. If someone else is able to take the strain – let it go!

Stop procrastinating

If you have things on your mind that you need to do – get them done! Dilly dallying will lead to an increase in stress as you rush to try and complete them when the deadline approaches.

Write things down

One way to handle stress is to write things down. When the brain is trying to remember things, it can be stressful in itself. The act of writing things down brings order to some people's thought processes and can consequently be calming.

Spend time with friends and family

Spending time with friends and family can help you get through stressful times.

It is thought that spending time socialising helps release Oxytocin, which is a natural stress reliever and it reduces the effect of cortisol.

Increase physical contact

Harder to do in the midst of a pandemic. But if you have people within your bubble, cuddling, kissing, hugging and sex can all help relieve stress.

Positive physical contact helps release oxytocin and lower cortisol. Consequently, lowering blood pressure and heart rate and reducing the fluttering feelings associated with stress and anxiety.

Spend time with a pet (or cuddle a baby!)

It has long been documented that stroking a pet can have an incredibly calming effect. Once again it is the caring interaction that is thought to release Oxytocin and counter the effects of stress.

Owning a pet can also give someone a sense of purpose, encourage exercise and providing companionship. However, owning a pet when you are unable to look after them properly can provoke additional stress and worry!

Take some Me Time

Take time out to do things that you really enjoy. This can be with friends or family, or on your own. But it is your choice as to how you would like to spend your time, not something you are doing to please someone else!

Challenge yourself! Learn a new skill or language or do something to stretch your abilities and gain a sense of satisfaction from completing it. The sense of achievement will contribute to your sense of wellbeing.

Laugh

Laughter has been shown to improve your immune system and mood, it relaxes your muscles and can lead to a feeling of well-being.

Herbal remedies – but check with your pharmacist to be sure they do not interact with any other prescription medication that you may be taking. Some of the following could also have side-effects.

Lemon balm: Lemon balm is a member of the mint family that is known for its soothing and anti-anxiety properties.

Omega-3 fatty acids: can potentially help.

Ashwagandha: Ashwagandha is an herb used in Ayurvedic medicine to treat stress and anxiety.

Green tea: Green tea contains many polyphenol antioxidants which provide health benefits. It is believed to lower stress and anxiety by increasing serotonin levels.

Valerian: Valerian root is often used to promote sleep. It contains valerenic acid, which alters gamma-aminobutyric acid (GABA) receptors, thought to reduce anxiety.

Kava kava: Kava kava is a member of the pepper family. The indigenous people of the South Pacific have long used it as a sedative; it is thought to be beneficial in reducing stress and anxiety.

Peppermint or chamomile teas both have soothing properties.

Aromatherapy

Using essential oils or burning a scented candle helps many people reduce feelings of stress and anxiety.

Some scents have been shown to be especially soothing.

Lavender – good for promoting sleep too

Rose

Vetiver

Bergamot

Roman chamomile

Neroli

Frankincense

Sandalwood

Ylang ylang

Orange or orange blossom

Geranium

Reduce your caffeine intake

Caffeine is a stimulant found in foods such as coffee, tea, chocolate and energy drinks. High doses can increase anxiety and make it harder to sleep.

Chew gum

Chewing gum is thought to relax tension in the jaw muscles and some studies have suggested that it increases blood flow to your brain.

Yoga

Yoga has become a popular method of stress relief and exercise and is helpful in promoting a feeling of calm wellbeing as well as improving your body's tone and flexibility.

Mindfulness

Mindfulness is a way of thinking, to reduce your mind wandering. It can be extremely helpful in reducing the anxiety-inducing effects of negative thinking.

Listen to soothing music

Listening to music can have a very relaxing effect on the body. Slow-paced instrumental music can help you feel more relaxed and help lower blood pressure, heart rate and reduce stress hormones.

Classical, Celtic, Native American and Indian music along with nature sounds, have all been shown to have particularly relaxing effects on the body. However listening to music you enjoy is also mood enhancing and relaxing.

The NHS recommends a selection of stress-relieving apps:

https://www.nhs.uk/apps-library/category/mental-health/

Work related stress:

All employers have a legal responsibility to look after their employees and do everything possible to ensure that the work or working practices do not adversely impact upon their employees' mental or physical health. When it is highlighted that a particular working practice or change in practice is affecting someone's health, businesses must ensure they are endeavouring to reduce or remove the impact.

The business is by no means culpable for all mental and physical illness that occurs whilst someone is employed. It is a fact that some employees will have pre-existing physical or mental health conditions when they join the business or may develop a mental or physical illness totally independently of any work-related cause.

Employers have further legal requirements, to make reasonable adjustments under equalities legislation and ensure there is no discrimination against an employee with any form of mental or physical illness or disability.

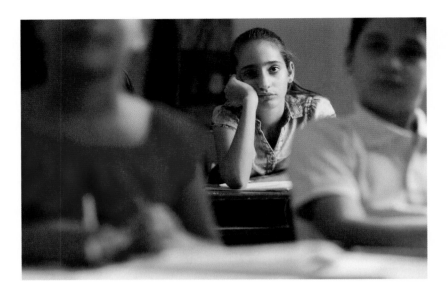

Help for parents, school staff, teachers, carers and friends of someone struggling with their mental health

Many children and young people struggle with their emotions and behaviour.

We know that the majority of mental health conditions start in early adolescence, but it can be really difficult to spot them early amidst all the confusion of puberty.

Around 20% of adolescents experience a mental health problem in any given year.

Often things start to become apparent at school, when they begin to experience problems with friends, family or schoolwork. They can become anxious, depressed, angry or scared and confused. This may just be a normal part of adolescence but could also be a sign that they are struggling with their mental wellbeing.

It is normal for life to have ups and downs, but when negative thoughts and feelings start to intrude, preventing young people from doing the things they would normally enjoy, or resulting in marked changes in their behaviour, they are likely to need help with their mental health.

Trust your instincts and if you think there could be something wrong, use the CARES approach to initiate a conversation.

Just as with a physical health condition, often there is no definite cause, there are a huge variety of factors can lead someone to struggle with their mental health.

Often people look to blame themselves for someone experiencing a mental health condition and desperately look for a cause. In your eyes they may have a charmed life with no cares or worries, do not judge, or reflect your opinions upon them.

Remember, this is about them, and getting them the right help when they need it.

The CARES Approach to Mental Health First Aid

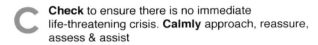

C **Check** to ensure there is no immediate life-threatening crisis. **Calmly** approach, reassure, assess & assist

A **Actively** Listen without judgment

R **Recommend** sources of immediate help – be particularly aware of signs of crisis

E **Encourage** to seek professional help

S **Suggest** possible self-help and other support options for better mental health

If there is a mental health problem emerging, or you believe a person could need help, help should be available. Often it is a relief for the young person to realise they don't have to help alone.

Professionals can support them with coping strategies to help manage the way that they are feeling and behaving.

Just as with physical health problems, diagnosing and treating a problem early can make things a lot easier.

Counselling and other advice services can help the child or young person talk about the way they are feeling and support them without making them feel judged.

The range of advice services for children and young people includes face-to-face counselling, one-to-one phone calls, webchat, email, forums and face-to-face sessions. There are also extremely helpful self-help forums, apps and online support.

Early intervention when someone is only just showing signs of struggling with their mental health can make a major difference to their recovery.

Prevention programmes and early intervention, such a parenting classes, family support, drug education, resilience programmes in schools, stress management, mental health awareness, have had a positive impact in reducing the numbers of people experiencing mental health crises.

Counselling and talking therapies

There are various talking therapies available and they are generally extremely helpful and effective.

Many schools, colleges and universities offer trained counselling services. Otherwise, their GP can refer to NHS counselling (although there may be a long wait)

Counselling is often recommended for young people who need additional support with a mental health disorder such as depression or eating disorders. The Counsellor will help them explore and address possible underlying problems and stress such as anxiety, bereavement, trauma, bullying, anger, relationships, low self-esteem and self-harm.

Counsellors can help young people better understand their feelings, identify what might be causing them to feel or behave a certain way and help them develop strategies to cope.

Medication can be prescribed to enhance mood, reduce anxiety, and reduce psychotic episodes. However, with all medication there is a risk benefit ratio and it is important to be aware of possible side-effects and ensure the medication is taken appropriately, avoiding possible drug interactions and contra-indications.

Some medication can affect sexual performance, or make your skin more prone to sunburn, they can affect your ability to drive, your mood and energy and ability to safely operate machinery at work.

All these factors need to be carefully considered and discussed before embarking on medication.

Psychological therapies: Talking with a mental health professional 1:1, or in a group session. For some people, these can be incredibly powerful. They are also accessible as apps, skype and zoom consultations, self-help books and courses. They are designed to help people gain self-help coping strategies, insight and find new ways of managing their condition.

There are numerous **complementary therapies** and **lifestyle changes** that can be prescribed by community health professionals or just accessed as self-help. Exercise and changes in diet, both have major roles to play in our mental health.

Support groups can be extremely helpful, MIND have a large online community Side By Side and access to many other support groups from their excellent website.

Rehabilitation programmes help people to re-build confidence and regain skills to be able to live independently.

Family, friends and work-colleagues will play an important role in someone's recovery.

Other professionals who can help:

The community health team:

GPs can offer a holistic approach to helping someone with a mental health issue. They can exclude any physical cause, explain how the disease might manifest itself and progress and prescribe medication and complementary therapies, through social prescribing networks.

Community psychiatric support and **psychologists** can also be helpful in supporting the person's recovery, along with other community support.

Counsellors, psychologists and psychotherapists: have also been proven to help people find new coping mechanisms with their illness. They offer various talking therapies that are specific to different conditions. Sometimes they focus on helping people cope with their conditions and sometimes the focus is more about problem solving, to assist them to solve stressful situations in their lives to cope better. This therapy can be conducted as 1:1 or in groups or families.

Psychiatrists: are medically trained doctors, specialising in treating mental illness. Their focus is usually more medication focussed and they would be more likely to see people with more complex or long-term conditions. Your GP can refer someone to a psychiatrist if they are experiencing more complex illness or are not responding to first line treatment. Although it is possible to access this help privately.

Mental health nurses: specially trained nurses focusing on caring for the mentally ill.

Occupational therapists: Can help re-train people and make appropriate workplace adjustments to help them return to work.

Care Co-ordinators – or key workers are community-based workers who co-ordinate care under the Care Programme Approach CPA and assist a multi-disciplinary team to communicate and work together to help the person cope in the community and workplace.

Different types of counselling

There are many different counselling options, but the following are the most commonly recommended for young people:

Some private psychotherapists work from home.

Family Therapy: This is inclusive therapy for the whole family. It can help improve family cohesion and the family counsellor can assist everyone in communicating more effectively and finding ways forward with areas of potential conflict. It is particularly helpful in addressing and assisting issues such as children's behavioural problems, family breakdown, addiction, abuse and domestic violence.

Cognitive Behavioural Therapy (CBT): CBT encourages people to think more positively about life, to review patterns of behaviour and try and change things to a positive spin. Typically, someone is offered 6 or 12 goal orientated weekly sessions. With practical homework in between.

Mindfulness: Mindfulness is often used alongside CBT and is effective at helping people to face difficult thoughts and feelings, rather than avoiding them, consequently this lessens their fear of them. Therapists often include meditation, yoga and breathing exercises. This combination can be extremely helpful.

Psychotherapy: This is conducted by a Psychotherapist, usually in a clinic or hospital. It is particularly helpful with long-term problems such as depression or eating disorders.

How to start the conversation:

1: Choose a good moment and be ready to help.

Calmly approach the person and assess the situation.

Choose a quiet room, where you won't be interrupted, where they will feel relaxed and more able to open up.

Respect their right not to want to discuss things. It could be because they are not ready to talk, it could be because they do not see you as the most appropriate person to open up to, or maybe they don't realise there is a problem, or possibly there has been a miscommunication and you have misread signs.

Carefully choose the best time and place to speak with them

Be sensitive and culturally aware – avoid doing anything that could offend, be misconstrued or could be considered culturally insensitive.

Don't be worried about asking them how they are feeling and how long they have been feeling this way.

2: Actively listen without judgement

This is the first step to someone recognising there may be a problem and that they might need help, is of vital importance. It is critical that they appreciate you are listening in a totally non-judgemental and confidential way and they can speak openly without any worry about prejudice, stigma or implications.

Try not to make assumptions, be patient and non-judgemental.

Never express any anger or disappointment or try to rationalise how they are feeling.

Think about your body language, where you are sitting and how you can make them feel most at ease.

It is important to ensure the person feels you are listening to them completely and concentrating on what they are saying.

Ensure you are not distracted or interrupted during this important communication.

Set-aside any pre-conceived judgements and ensure you listen to them with a completely open mind.

Use verbal and non-verbal listening and communication skills to ensure that the person knows you are actively listening to them and engaging in what they are saying.

Do not be tempted to interrupt them or to suggest how they may be feeling.

Empathise through gestures and body language.

Accept what they are saying, even if it doesn't make sense from your perspective.

Try not to jump in and offer solutions.

Never give examples of someone else with similar problems as that is seriously breaching confidentiality and will dent their trust and confidence in you too.

Clarify and repeat back what they have told you, so you are both sure you have understood and summarised the situation properly.

3. Recommend sources of immediate help

Once they have felt they have been listened to and better understood, they may be more receptive to you offering further support and information.

Make it clear you recognise how they are feeling and explain how you can help them to get help and start feeling better.

See if there is any obvious practical help that can be sorted to help ease their stress. For example, if they are overwhelmed with school work or exam stress, there may be a way school can help.

Be ready to support them making an appointment to see their GP – they may or may not feel more comfortable with someone coming with them.

Be ready to signpost them to additional support, providing the time is right and they are not too overwhelmed with their current distress.

It is extremely courageous of them to open up to you and not an easy thing to do. They are likely to feel worried and vulnerable and uncertain as to whether there are any negative implications to the conversation. Reassure them, thank them for confiding and explain, they are not alone – 1 in 4 people experience these feelings and you are here to help.

4. Encourage to seek professional help

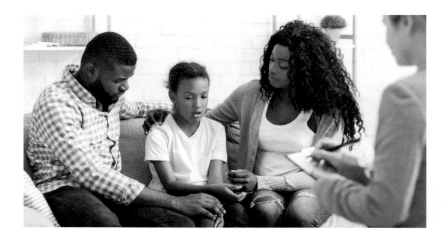

Someone with a mental health issue will generally recover faster with appropriate professional help.

Exploring possible options together and be ready to allay fears of possible stigma, or mistaken beliefs about various options.

Helping them realise that they are not suffering alone, can be empowering for them. They may not have known about possible options; including counselling, psychological therapy, medication, financial support, help for family members, specific support groups. They may not have even realised why they were feeling as they were.

Ask if there is anyone else (such as a friend, family member, teacher, other trusted adult) who they would like to tell who might be able to offer additional support to them.

Their GP – can offer ongoing holistic support and treatment and refer to appropriate professionals as necessary. They will also be able to rule out medical reasons for the way the person is feeling.

Crisis Line – they may have already been given the Crisis Line number. If so there will be a trained healthcare professional who should be able to help them.

Samaritans – 116 123 – open 24 hours a day, 365 days a year. With trained operators ready to help.

Call NHS 111 or 999 if seriously worried that they are a risk to themselves or others.

Reasons to contact the emergency services:

The person is experiencing serious suicidal thoughts or feelings

They are thinking or talking about harming themselves or someone else

Experiencing acute medical symptoms

They have already hurt themselves

You feel threatened by their behaviour and our worried that in approaching you could aggravate the situation and put yourself, or them at greater risk.

Please note: It is vital to respect the person's consent. They cannot be forced to seek help or to go to A&E. It is quite common for people to periodically have suicidal thoughts, but not to act on them.

5. Suggest possible self-help options for better mental health

Explain available self-help strategies

Let them know about specific support groups

Encourage them to discuss how they are feeling with other close friends and family

Signpost to appropriate community and voluntary sector organisations, there are online communities and peer support networks. All there to help. MIND is a superb website to explore together.

Look at proven self-help coping mechanisms

Respect the person's wishes if they prefer to seek culturally-based care.

MIND has some excellent resources to help someone experiencing a mental health issue https://www.mind.org.uk/information-support/helping-someone-else/ and a huge range of specific topics for the person experiencing the mental health issue to access themselves https://www.mind.org.uk/information-support/.

Young Minds also has a wealth of resources.

Getting help:

Your GP is often the first port of call. Be open to all suggested options.

If the first thing they try doesn't work, encourage them to look at alternatives. Sometimes the first counsellor may not have quite the right approach or be the best person to help. Support the young person in gaining alternative help – they deserve it.

Sometimes online support or group therapy may be the best approach. They should have a say as to what works best for them.

The Royal College of Psychiatrists have produced information specifically for children and young people to help them get the support they need U can cope! .

Once you have had the initial conversation, things you can do to support them:

1. Try not to change how you behave towards them. Retain boundaries and consistency – this keeps a level of control and stability in their life.

2. However, be sensitive to changes in their mood. If they are not feeling their best, ensure you are ready to further talk if they wish to.

3. Arrange a time and place that is stress-free for both of you, ensure you will have enough time to have a proper conversation without being interrupted.

4. Be calm and positive.

5. They may have been very worried that someone won't understand, your continuing support will mean a great deal.

6. It is important to reinforce that you care about them, are there for them and will do whatever you can to support them in getting the help they need.

7. Make it clear that everything they tell you will remain confidential. **Never** break this confidence (unless you have a significant concern for their safety).

8. However, encourage them to think about other people that might be safe and helpful to confide in (e.g. other family members, a teacher, trusted adult, carer, friend, GP, helpline).

9. Suggest moderated self-help groups, these can be really helpful to talk things through with others with similar experiences.

10. Be ready to help with practical support, such as taking them to appointments, even if you wait outside.

If they are referred to CAMHS (Child and Adolescent Mental Health), the team will try and include the family if appropriate and helpful. Parents and carers can also ask CAMHS staff questions at any point in the assessment or treatment.

Parents Guide To Support A-Z – Young Mind's excellent resource

Finding further help:

The NHS Mental Health Team are overstretched. If the child or young person does not fit the criteria for CAMHS, your GP may be able to suggest alternative local counselling provision for young people.

Schools, colleges and universities can also refer young people to CAMHS. In addition, they may offer their own counsellor or mental health services on-site.

There are many charities and other organisations out there offering advice, support and solidarity from helplines, group forums and message boards, email- webchat- text- and email services.

Counsellors and therapists also operate privately:

British Association for Counselling and Psychotherapy (BACP)

- Professional body that sets standards for therapeutic practice, and provides information for therapists, clients of therapy, and the general public. Their helpful website includes information about counselling and psychotherapy and how to find the right therapist.

- Phone: 01455 883 300 (Mon-Fri 09:00 – 17:00)

Association of Child Psychotherapists

- This is a register of accredited Child and Adolescent Psychotherapists in the UK.

Counselling Directory

- Lists private counsellors and psychotherapists registered with a professional body. They can also provide information on the different types of talking therapies including family therapy.

British Psychological Society

- Has information on how psychologists can help with mental health problems, and how to find a psychologist.

Youth Wellbeing Directory

- Lists local services for young people's mental health and wellbeing.

Counselling for families - Relate

Support, guidance and counselling services for families and young people. When families are going through a tough time, relate offers support to help everyone settle. Phone: 0300 100 1234 or contact your local Relate Centre.

- Relate (for families)

- Relate (for family life and parenting)

- Relate (parenting teenagers)

- Relate counselling options: Live chatroom, message a counsellor, webcam counselling, telephone counselling

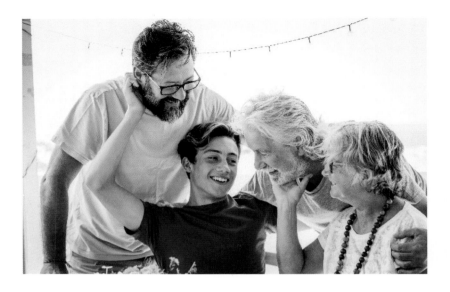

Building resilience:

Resilience is our ability to cope with life's ups and downs. It has been shown that there are recognised steps that we can all take that can boost our ability to deal with pressure and reduce the adverse impact of stress on our lives. Resilience is the ability to adapt to challenging circumstances without it taking too large an impact on our mental well-being.

FIVE STEPS TO MENTAL WELLBEING

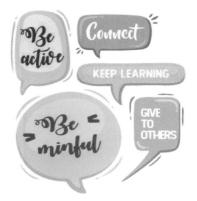

This is what the NHS recommends based on evidence and research.

We can improve our wellbeing by building these five steps into our day-to-day lives.

If you give them a try, you may feel happier, more positive and able to get the most from life.

Simple changes can make a big difference:

Be assertive

Calmly, clearly and politely let people know if you believe they are being unreasonable or exerting undue pressure on you. Say no to things, if you feel overwhelmed. Be assertive in your approach, seek additional support if necessary.

Resolve conflict, if you can. Although extremely difficult, facing up to issues can help everyone find ways to move forward.

It isn't always the case, but there should be a supportive structure at work. Your line manager, human resources (HR) department, union representatives, or employee assistance schemes – should be there for you. Stress is not a sign of weakness.

Additional resources can be found:

Time to Change's resources on stress, depression and mental health support at work

Health and Safety Executive's information on work-related stress

At university or college, there should be support available from student services, your tutors, or the student union.

Close family and friends can often offer great non-judgemental love and support.

Relaxation techniques can be helpful.

Take time out for yourself and do some of the things that promote a feeling of relaxation and well-being.

Some people find a country walk, exercise, having a bath, listening to music and a wealth of other things – work well for them to help restore their mental health.

Identify what works for you and schedule time in your diary to make it happen.

Learn a new skill, hobby or take up a specific interest

When people feel stressed, they often feel exhausted and don't want to make the effort to socialise or do new things. Pushing yourself to try something new or to pursue a hobby you enjoy can be extremely therapeutic and can also be a good way to meet new people.

Reconnect with friends

More than just on Facebook, pick up the phone, or meet them for a walk or cup of tea. Spending time with other people usually makes people feel better. However, if you are feeling a little vulnerable, select the friends you meet with carefully, some friends can be needy and a drain on your energy, it is not those you need at the moment, spend time instead with people that boost your mood. Chatting to friends about the things you are struggling with can help give a sense of perspective – and it works both ways too! It has been proven that laughing and smiling is contagious and releases hormones that help you feel better too.

Look carefully at your work, life, family balance and make yourself more me time!

It is easy to lose your identity in the business of life when working, or as a spouse, partner, parent or child – try and establish your own identity and carve time out for yourself. Sometimes it feels impossible and selfish to try and take time for yourself. However, it is critical and everyone will benefit in the long-term.

Be kind to yourself and don't stress about being stressed!!

Forgive yourself if you feel you have made a mistake, or don't live up to your own high expectations. Try to remember that nobody's perfect and putting additional pressure on yourself doesn't help.

Do things that give you a sense of achievement

Set yourself small, achievable goals and celebrate your achievements.

Work smarter not harder:

Without procrastinating, try and establish what things can wait, or someone else can do. This will take some of the pressure off you. The saying is that if you want something done, you should ask a busy person! However, everyone has their limits and when the busy person says no, other people step up – or things simply might not happen!

Ensure you are caring for your physical health too

Our mental and physical health are often inextricably linked. If we begin to feel run down, we often feel more lethargic and less able to do things and this takes its health on our mental well-being too.

Sleep

Sleep enables the body and mind to rest and heal. Getting enough sleep is critical. It is often a vicious circle - stress can often make it difficult to sleep, but lack of sleep makes it harder for you to cope with stress.

Exercise

Whatever your capabilities, it is vital to be active. Being physically active boosts our physical and mental health. Start with small lifestyle changes, even a short walk or some gently gardening can begin to boost your mood.

Sunlight and being outside makes us feel better.

Eat healthily

When busy or stressed, it is tempting to skip meals or crave sweet, starchy food. There is a proven link between having a healthy diet and physical and mental well-being.

Get away

Take a break or holiday. Time away from your normal routine can help you relax and feel refreshed. Even spending a day in a different place can help you feel more able to face stress.

Remember you don't have to cope with it alone – a problem shared is often a problem put into perspective.

Mind have helpful resources https://www.mind.org.uk/information-support/types-of-mental-health-problems/stress/developing-resilience/#collapsef06cf

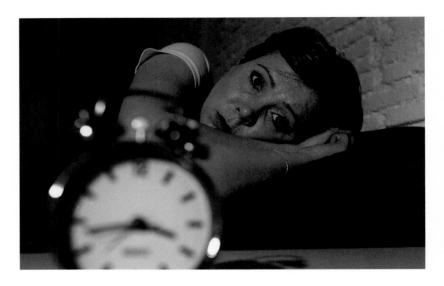

Insomnia

Severe insomnia can wreak havoc with mental health and physical wellbeing. The NHS define insomnia as regularly experiencing problems sleeping. Sleep is incredibly important and enables the body and mind to relax and reboot, rest and heal. Getting enough sleep is critical. It is often a vicious circle – stress can often make it difficult to sleep, but lack of sleep makes it harder for you to cope with stress. Insomnia often hits people at different stages in their lives and increased stress, worry or sorrow can adversely impact upon our sleep patterns. Often children struggle sleeping around exam time, new parents exist on ridiculously disrupted sleep and again it is something that can cause problems as people get older and are affected by the menopause or an increasing need to go to the loo at night. Sometimes people have prolonged periods without sleep for no apparent reason! Often simple changes to sleeping habits can help. Here we offer some handy tips for understanding and dealing with insomnia, as well as improving your general mental health.

What is insomnia?

You have insomnia if you regularly:

- find it hard to go to sleep

- wake up several times during the night

- lie awake at night

- wake up early and cannot go back to sleep

- still feel tired after waking up

- find it hard to nap during the day even though you feel tired

- feel tired and irritable during the day

- find it difficult to concentrate during the day because of tiredness

Many people experience these symptoms for months, sometimes years.

How much sleep do you need?

Everyone needs different amounts of sleep. On average, we need:

- adults: 7 to 9 hours

- children: 9 to 13 hours

- toddlers and babies: 12 to 17 hours

You probably do not get enough sleep if you're constantly tired during the day.

Do you have a sleep problem?

Most people experience problems with sleep in their life. In fact, it's thought that a third of people experience episodes of insomnia at some point.

What causes insomnia?

Insomnia can be triggered by physical and psychological conditions (such as depression or anxiety) or a combination of both. The most common causes are:

- stress, anxiety or depression

- noise

- new baby

- a room that's too hot or cold

- uncomfortable beds

- alcohol, caffeine or nicotine

- recreational drugs like cocaine or ecstasy

- jet lag

- shift work

- working too late into the evening and being unable to switch off

- worries, excitement and things playing on your mind

- pregnancy

- needing to get up in the night to go to the loo

- hormonal changes from menopause

- some foods

- underlying medical conditions

- Side effects from some medications

How you can treat insomnia yourself?

Insomnia can often be helped by changing your sleeping habits.

Do:

- go to bed and wake up at the same time every day – only go to bed when you feel tired

- relax at least 1 hour before bed – for example, take a bath or read a book

- make sure your bedroom is dark and quiet – use thick curtains, blinds, an eye mask or ear plugs

- exercise regularly during the day

- make sure your mattress, pillows and covers are comfortable

- often a milky drink before bedtime can help – or getting one in the night, if you can't sleep

Do not:

- smoke or drink alcohol, tea or coffee at least 6 hours before going to bed

- eat a big meal late at night

- exercise at least 4 hours before bed

- watch television or use devices right before going to bed – the bright light makes you more awake and working late into the evening can leave you feeling pre-occupied

- nap during the day

- drive when you feel sleepy

- sleep in after a bad night's sleep – stick to your regular sleeping hours instead

Avoiding the blue light of electronic devices is critical. Scrolling through content, surfing the web, looking at emails or playing games will activate the brain, just when it should be relaxing. Blue wavelength light from computers, tablets and mobile phones has been shown to disrupt the production of the sleep hormone, melatonin. We need melatonin to regulate our circadian rhythms and feel sleepy at bed-time.

Therefore, people suffering from insomnia should avoid using digital devices at least 90 minutes before planning to go to sleep.

Should I see a Doctor?

Insomnia should never be treated in A&E. Your pharmacist may be able to help. You can get herbal medication and various mild sleeping sedatives from a pharmacy. But they will not get rid of your insomnia and could have many side effects. Sleeping pills can often make you drowsy the next day. You might find it hard to get things done. You should not drive the day after taking them. See a GP if:

- changing your sleeping habits has not worked

- you have had trouble sleeping for a prolonged amount of time

- your insomnia is affecting your daily life in a way that makes it hard for you to cope

A GP will try to find out what is causing your insomnia so you get the right treatment. A GP can carry out an evaluation including a physical exam and a sleep history. They will first look to exclude any common medical conditions that might be preventing your sleep. Keeping a sleep diary for one or two weeks can be invaluable. Sometimes they may refer you to a specialist sleep centre. Sometimes you'll be referred to a therapist for cognitive behavioural therapy (CBT). This can help you change the thoughts and behaviours that keep you from sleeping. GPs now rarely prescribe sleeping pills to treat insomnia. Sleeping pills can have serious side effects and you can become dependent on them. Sleeping pills should only be prescribed for a few days, or weeks at the most, if:

- your insomnia is seriously debilitating

- other treatments have not worked

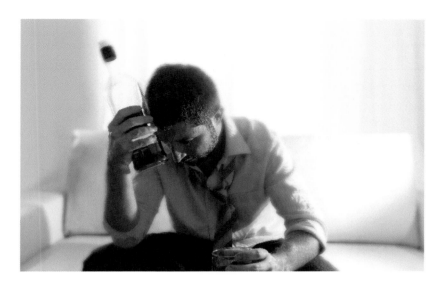

Substance Misuse – Drugs and alcohol

"Substance abuse (or misuse) refers to the harmful or hazardous use of psychoactive substances, including alcohol and illicit drugs" – WHO definition.

Unfortunately, many people try to escape stress or unhappiness by turning to and misusing substances such as drugs and alcohol. This can swiftly descend into a downward spiral of interdependence and makes any underlying mental health problems far harder to treat.

Sometimes it is drug or alcohol dependence that leads to mental health disorders. We know there are strong links between the use of various drugs and mental health disorders and often alcohol abuse leads to depression and vice versa. Alcohol and other drugs actually affect the chemistry in the brain and can exacerbate mental health disorders.

When someone has drug or alcohol dependence combined with a mental health disorder, this means they have a dual diagnosis which can lead to more serious mental health problems.

Drugs can be divided into 4 main categories:

- Stimulants – e.g., cocaine, ecstasy etc

- Opiates – e.g., heroin, codeine etc

- Depressants – e.g., alcohol, cannabis etc

- Hallucinogens – e.g., LSD, magic mushrooms etc

Alcohol misuse

Alcohol misuse is defined as regularly drinking more than the 'lower-risk limits' of alcohol consumption as recommended by the NHS.

Regularly drinking more than 14 units of alcohol a week.

If you do drink as much as 14 units a week and have difficulty cutting down, it is better to spread this evenly over 3 or more days, rather than to binge-drink it in one or 2 sessions.

Dangers of drinking alcohol whilst taking prescribed medications:

Alcohol can reduce the effectiveness of some medications, as and may intensify possible side effects. Always read the leaflet with the medication before taking it and adhere to any advised precautions, such as avoiding alcohol.

Drugs and alcohol and how they affect your mental health

Both tend to affect the way you perceive things, they alter your behaviour, mental and physical health, both in the short term – when experiencing the highs and lows and in the longer term. These effects differ from person to person and can also fluctuate for an individual depending on who they are with, how much they have eaten, whether they are dehydrated, their mood and many other moderating factors.

Short term effects include:

- Reduction or removal of inhibitions

- Violent, abusive or provocative behaviour

- Impaired judgement

- Anxiety, paranoia and depression – including suicidal thoughts

- Confusion, memory problems

- Altered perception of reality

Alcohol and drug consumption can make the treatment of common physical first aid emergencies more difficult:

Alcohol and drug ingestion can make it harder to help in a physical first aid emergency. Often someone who is drunk or high is less compliant and may even be confrontational and violent. This can make it extremely difficult to help them.

If someone has hit their head, it is more difficult to assess the extent of any injury.

When someone has consumed large amounts of alcohol, it affects their ability to maintain their body heat. Consequently, they may end up experiencing hypothermia. Hypothermia affects the stability of your heart and makes you more prone to a heart attack, it also affects the ability for your blood to clot and so bleeding is more difficult to control.

Helping someone you think has problems with drug or alcohol misuse:

Do not try and have a meaningful conversation with them whilst they are seriously under the influence of drugs or alcohol. They may not remember your conversation, or it could promote an unwelcome reaction.

If they are under the influence, it is their physical well-being that is the priority:

Ensure they are safe.

If they are unconscious or losing consciousness – put them into the recovery position to keep their airway clear.

If they are outside, or in a cold environment and have drunk too much – keep them warm.

If they have taken drugs and appear to be over-heating, try and encourage them to drink regular sips of water.

If they are having trouble breathing or expressing suicidal thoughts – call the emergency services.

We have all seen tricky situations happen or been involved in confrontational situations ourselves, where someone looks like they need help, but we are frightened to get involved because of the aggressive or strange way the person is behaving. This may be caused by the abuse of drugs and alcohol.

Common causes of threatening or confrontational behaviour

The person may be behaving strangely for many reasons: they could be angry, high on drugs and alcohol, or suffering from side effects of prescription medication.

In older people, infections are often the underlying cause of confusion. It is therefore important that these possibilities are investigated if someone rapidly becomes confused and disorientated.

They could also be suffering from brain trauma, have had a stroke, be confused (possibly due to any number of reasons), mentally ill, be having a life crisis.

It is also possible you have misunderstood the context of the situation and don't have all the information about it. Perhaps all is not as it seems.

Whatever the cause of confrontational or worrying behaviour, if you feel uncomfortable, stay well back and contact the emergency services and give them all the information you have.

The most important advice is never put yourself at risk and always trust your instincts.

First aid for someone who has collapsed from excess alcohol.

Ensure you have the skills to look after someone who has collapsed following too much alcohol. It is absolutely vital that if someone is unconscious and unable to maintain their own airway, that you put them into the recovery position. In addition, someone should stay with them to ensure they do not asphyxiate on their tongue or vomit.

When someone has consumed so much alcohol that they have collapsed, immediately check that they are breathing and then roll them into the recovery position. This should help to ensure their airway remains clear.

If someone is drunk, it becomes harder for them to maintain their body temperature and they can quickly succumb to hypothermia.

If they are outside, bring them in. Alternatively, if you are unable to move them, insulate them from the ground and cover them with a coat or blanket.

Keep checking they are breathing and that their airway remains clear, especially if they are vomiting.

The effects of alcohol can also make it harder to assess serious signs and symptoms.

When someone who is drunk bumps their head, a medical professional should always check them. Someone should monitor anyone with a serious head injury for the next 48 hours to check for any signs of brain injury. This is even more important if they have been drinking or have taken any other substances.

Mental Health First Aid for drug and alcohol misuse using CARES

– A mental health first aid action plan:

Check for immediate life-threatening emergency. Calmly approach, reassure, assess & assist.

Actively listen without judgment

Recommend sources of immediate help – be particularly aware of signs of crisis

Encourage to seek professional help

Suggest possible self-help and other support options for better mental health

Having established that there is no immediate life-threatening emergency:

Calmly approach them and reassuringly try to help.

Choose a quiet room, where you won't be interrupted, where they will feel relaxed and more able to open up.

Respect their right not to want to discuss things. It could be because they are not ready to talk, it could be because they do not see you as the most appropriate person to open up to, or maybe they don't realise there is a problem, or possibly there has been a miscommunication and you have misread signs.

Actively listen without judgment

Try not to make assumptions, be patient and non-judgemental.

Think about your body language, where you are sitting and how you can make them feel most at ease.

Maintain eye contact.

Try to establish the nature of the problem and what they are taking or have taken.

This information will be extremely helpful to the emergency services if they were to require emergency first aid.

Recommend sources of immediate help – be particularly aware of signs of crisis

The very first step is to acknowledge that there is a problem. Then talking to friends and family may be the next course of action.

Encourage them to seek professional help.

Visiting their GP is usually the best initial healthcare professional.

GPs will be able to further signpost them to additional NHS drug and alcohol treatment services such as cognitive and behavioural therapy, detox and medication.

Suggest possible self-help and other support options for better mental health – see the specific resources section at the back of the book.

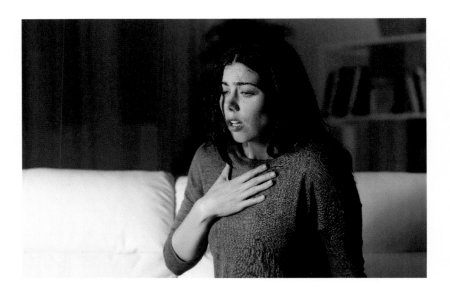

Anxiety Disorders

Everybody experiences anxiety at some point in their life. Anxiety can be a helpful, natural response that helps us avoid dangerous situations and find solutions to problems. Anxiety can vary in severity from a sense of unease, to an overwhelming panic. Panic attacks can be so severe that they can lead people to think they are having a heart attack or dying.

Common symptoms of anxiety can include all the systems of the body:

- Cardiac effects such as: palpitations, chest pain, flushing and a rapid heart beat

- Respiratory problems: hyperventilation, breathlessness

- Neurological: dizziness, headache, sweating, tingling and numbness, dry mouth, tremor

- Gastrointestinal and renal: nausea, vomiting, diarrhoea, gagging and choking

- Musculoskeletal: muscle aches and pains (in particular tension in the neck, shoulders and lower back) restlessness

- Urinary – frequently needing to pee

Psychological effects include:

- Excessive or unrealistic fears and worries about all aspects of life

- Decreasing concentration and struggling with memory

- Difficulty making decisions

- Irritability, confusion and anger for no apparent reason, or out of proportion to the provocation

- Restlessness and inability to settle

- Tiredness, disturbed sleep and vivid dreams

- Intrusive thoughts

- Confusion

Behavioural effects:

- Repetitive, compulsive behaviour – checking things multiple times

- Uncomfortable in social situations, actively avoiding social interaction

- Phobic behaviour – leading someone to want to escape from uncomfortable situations

Some medical professionals frequently use the Goldberg Anxiety Scale to assess how severely someone's life is impacted by their anxiety.

Anxiety can be experienced in many different ways and at different levels and can also be diagnosed as specific anxiety disorders.

Some commonly diagnosed anxiety disorders are:

- **Generalised anxiety disorder (GAD)** – this means having regular or uncontrollable worries about many different things. This tends to be a broad diagnosis, that encompasses a wide range of different experiences.

- **Social anxiety disorder** – this diagnosis means someone experiences extreme fear or anxiety triggered by social situations (such as parties, workplaces, or any social situation). It is also known as social phobia.

- **Panic disorder** –having regular or frequent panic attacks without a clear cause or trigger. Experiencing panic disorder can make someone constantly afraid of having another panic attack, to the point that this fear itself can trigger panic attacks.

- **Phobias** – a phobia is an extreme fear or anxiety triggered by a particular situation (such as social situations) or a particular object (such as spiders).

- **Post-traumatic stress disorder (PTSD)** – this is a diagnosis if someone develops anxiety problems after going through something traumatic. PTSD can cause flashbacks or nightmares which can cause the person to re-live all the fear and anxiety experienced during the actual event.

- **Obsessive-compulsive disorder (OCD)** – anxiety problems involving repetitive thoughts, behaviours or urges.

- **Health anxiety** –obsessions and compulsions relating to illness, including researching symptoms or checking to see if they have them. It is related to OCD.

- **Body dysmorphic disorder (BDD)** –obsessions and compulsions relating to physical appearance.

- **Perinatal anxiety or perinatal OCD** – some women develop anxiety problems during pregnancy or in the first year after giving birth.

It is extremely common to experience anxiety alongside other mental health problems, such as depression or suicidal feelings.

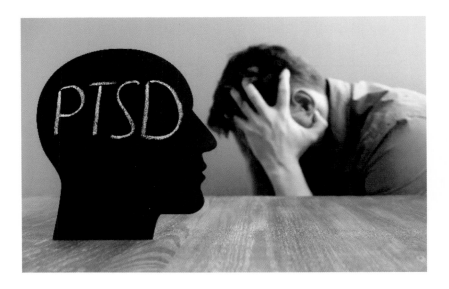

Post-Traumatic Stress Disorder (PTSD)

Anyone can experience post-traumatic stress from something distressing that they have seen, experienced or that has happened to someone close to them.

It is perfectly normal to feel any of the following after a traumatic event:

- Elation/an adrenaline buzz

- Anger

- Confusion

- Flashbacks and bad dreams

- Depression

Generally, it is advised, that if a person is experiencing the following symptoms four or more weeks after a trauma, seeking professional help should be encouraged. However, if you think they need professional help sooner than this, please don't wait.

Symptoms that could indicate someone may be developing PTSD, if they are still apparent weeks after the event:

1. they remain very upset or fearful.

2. continue to experience intense, ongoing feelings of distress.

3. begin to withdraw from family or friends and avoid social situations.

4. have ongoing trauma-related nightmares and feel jumpy or on edge.

5. continually obsessing about the trauma.

6. have lost their enjoyment in life.

7. Have intrusive thoughts, feelings or sensations that are interfering with usual activities.

If you are unsure if you or a loved one is experiencing PTSD or are worried about their welfare, talk to a health professional.

MIND offer the following tips on coping with flashbacks

Flashbacks can be very distressing, but there are things you can do that might help. You could:

Focus on your breathing. When you are frightened, you might stop breathing normally. This increases feelings of fear and panic, so it can help to concentrate on breathing slowly in and out while counting to five.

Carry an object that reminds you of the present. Some people find it helpful to touch or look at a particular object during a flashback. This might be something you decide to carry in your pocket or bag, or something that you have with you anyway, such as a keyring or a piece of jewellery.

Tell yourself that you are safe. It may help to tell yourself that the trauma is over and you are safe now. It can be hard to think in this way during a flashback, so it could help to write down or record some useful phrases at a time when you're feeling better.

Comfort yourself. For example, you could curl up in a blanket, cuddle a pet, listen to soothing music or watch a favourite film.

Keep a diary. Making a note of what happens when you have a flashback could help you spot patterns in what triggers these experiences for you. You might also learn to notice early signs that they are beginning to happen.

Try grounding techniques. Grounding techniques can keep you connected to the present and help you cope with flashbacks or intrusive thoughts. For example, you could describe your surroundings out loud or count objects of a particular type or colour.

Flashback triggers:

Some people find certain experiences, situations or people seem to trigger flashbacks or other symptoms. These might include specific reminders of past trauma, such as smells, sounds, words, places or particular types of books, films or gaming. Some dates or anniversaries may be particularly difficult for people as well.

The key advice following trauma is to:

Speak when you are ready to; for some people telling everyone is helpful, for others they need time and may need a long time before they are ready to share their experience.

Be kind to yourself and understand that your mind will take time to heal too.

There are some extremely helpful and supportive organisations listed in the resource section at the back of this book.

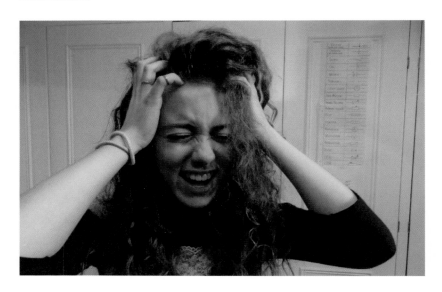

Panic attacks

Panic attacks are a form of fear response. They are an exaggeration of your body's normal response to danger, stress or excitement – the fight, flight or fright response.

Recognising someone could be having a panic attack:

Someone experiencing a panic attack could experience any of the following:

- a pounding or racing heartbeat

- feeling faint, dizzy or light-headed

- feeling very hot or very cold

- sweating, trembling or shaking

- nausea (feeling sick)

- pain in the chest or abdomen

- struggling to breathe or feeling like they are choking

- shaky legs or jelly legs

- a total disconnect from their mind, body or surroundings

During a panic attack the person may appear petrified that they are:

- losing control or going mad

- going to faint

- having a heart attack

- going to die.

Panic attacks can happen during the day or night. Some people only ever experience one panic attack; others have them regularly, or several in a short space of time.

Most panic attacks last between 5–20 minutes and can come on very quickly. Symptoms will usually peak within 10 minutes but can continue for longer.

It is extremely important that a Mental Health First Aider does not automatically assume that the person is experiencing a panic attack. The CARES approach is a great way to help:

Check for life-threatening problems. **C**almly approach, reassure, assess & assist.

Actively Listen without judgment

Recommend sources of immediate help – be particularly aware of signs of crisis

Encourage to seek professional help

Suggest possible self-help and other support options for better mental health

It is vital that the first aider remains as calm as possible in order to avoid aggravating the situation.

They should initially give first aid to help the person experiencing the panic attack.

Do not automatically assume that the person is experiencing a panic attack, unless it is extremely obvious that is the problem. The signs and symptoms of angina or a heart attack can be extremely similar to that of a panic attack. People who experience regular panic attacks may also experience a heart attack!

If you suspect someone may be having a heart attack – help them to sit in the lazy W position, supported against a wall.

- Ask if they have felt like this before. Have they been prescribed anything to help?

- If they have a history of angina and have been prescribed a GTN tablet or spray – help them to take it according to prescribed instructions, sprayed or place under their tongue.

- Tablets – 1 tablet under your tongue as soon as possible. If still in pain after 5 minutes they can have a second dose by putting 1 more tablet under your tongue. If still in pain after 5 minutes give a third and final dose.

- Spray – 1 or 2 sprays under your tongue. Can be repeated as above

- Do not use more than 3 doses during an angina attack. 1 dose is either 1 tablet or 1 to 2 sprays.

- If the GTN spray doesn't help and they have been prescribed a 300mg aspirin, they should take it now. Ideally this should be chewed.

- Phone for an ambulance, keep them as calm as possible.

- Get an AED if available and be ready to give CPR if they lose consciousness and stop breathing.

It can also be difficult to distinguish a serious panic attack from an asthma attack – particularly if the person is asthmatic. Struggling for breath during an asthma attack can trigger a panic attack. Ensure you have the skills to help someone experiencing an asthma attack.

Panic Attacks: How to Help

Panic attacks can happen to anyone, without any obvious cause or warning. They can be extremely alarming both for the person experiencing the attack and anyone trying to help

Exams increase stress – and children and teenagers up and down the country will be sitting in exams halls, waiting to hear the famous words "you can turn your papers over now". For some, exams cause no problems at all, many just get butterflies, but for some, the fear of exams can result in full blown panic attacks.

Certain times of life can make people more prone to panic attacks, often those going through the menopause experience them and early Alzheimer's can also result in a higher incidence. Increased stress and overload can often be a contributory factor. However, there does not need to be any obvious reason – sometimes, they just happen!

Panic is an extreme feeling of fear and dread, and usually the overwhelming desire to escape an uncomfortable situation. Most people have experienced a sense of panic at some time in their life – it is a perfectly normal response. Some people have a history of panic attacks and know what can trigger them. For others, they can occur suddenly, with no obvious cause.

Physical reactions may be frightening and can include the following:

- A pounding and racing heart or even palpitations (feeling your heart is stopping or missing beats)

- Shortness of breath or a feeling of choking

- Shaking, tingling or numbness in your fingers and toes

- Feeling sick and dizzy

- Sweating

- Needing the loo

- Thinking you might die

- Feeling you are losing control of your mind – even that you are going crazy

- Aggressiveness, sometimes due to the wish to escape

- Difficulty breathing due to panic attacks should not be confused with asthma.

Asthma:

Asthma is an extremely common chronic and potentially life-threatening condition. When someone has Asthma; their airways go into spasm which causes tightness of the chest; the linings of the airways become inflamed and produce phlegm leading to severe difficulty in breathing.

If someone is having an asthma attack, they need their medication and help quickly, whereas panic attacks are usually short lived, and the casualty quickly makes a full recovery.

During asthma attacks, casualties wheeze, struggling to breathe out, whereas large volumes of air can be heard entering and leaving the lungs when someone is hyperventilating and having a panic attack.

If someone is having a panic attack:

- Reassure them; they may be unable to explain what has caused them to panic and do not pressure them to do this, your calm presence should help.

- Speak to them in positive, supportive terms – "you will be okay, this will pass in a minute" etc.

During a panic attack:

- **Encourage them to focus on their breathing.** It can help to concentrate on breathing slowly in and out while counting to five.

- **Stamp on the spot.** Some people find this helps control their breathing.

- **Try grounding techniques.** Grounding techniques can help someone feel more in control. They are especially useful if experiencing dissociation (a feeling of disconnect or flashbacks) during panic attacks.

- Ask them to concentrate on sounds around them.

- Try walking barefoot.

- Wrapping themselves in a blanket and feeling it around them.

- Touching something or sniffing something with a strong smell.

- Focus on the sensations right now. Some people keep a box of things with different textures and smells (for example perfume, a blanket and some smooth stones) ready for when they need it.

- Remove them from anything obviously causing distress.

- Encourage them to breathe calmly and slowly, in and out through their nose and out of their mouth, to reduce the amount of carbon dioxide being lost.

- Small sips of water may help to calm them.

- If symptoms get worse, get medical help.

- When the panic attack is over, talk it through with them. Discuss relaxation techniques and other helpful means of coping in case this happens again.

Paper bags:

Do **not** suggest breathing in and out of a paper bag. People used to think breathing in and out of a paper bag was helpful during a panic attack, and the physiology makes sense; breathing out in panic results in the loss of carbon dioxide in the blood and breathing into a bag restores the lost CO2.

The danger with a paper bag is that the casualty may become dependent upon it and can panic if they do not have one to hand (my mother suffered from numerous panic attacks in the early stages of her Alzheimers and quickly became obsessed with paper bags after someone had encouraged her to use one).

It is extremely dangerous using a paper bag with someone who is having an asthma attack; this can make things worse.

If attacks are persistent and severe, the patient can be referred for specialist help.

There are some really helpful contacts for anxiety listed in the resource section at the back of this book.

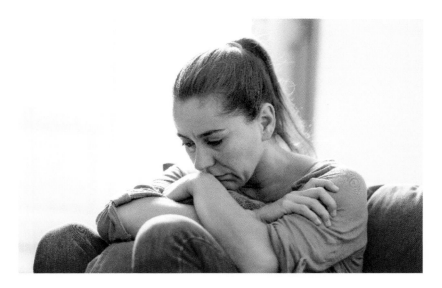

Depression

The NHS explains that: "Depression is more than simply feeling unhappy or fed up for a few days.

Most people go through periods of feeling down, but when you are depressed you feel persistently sad for weeks or months, rather than just a few days.

Some people think depression is trivial and not a genuine health condition. They are wrong – it is a real illness with real symptoms. Depression is not a sign of weakness or something you can "snap out of" by "pulling yourself together".

The good news is that with the right treatment and support, most people with depression can make a full recovery."

When people acknowledge they are depressed and find the right treatment (self-help or professional help) – they can begin to feel far better and go on to recover fully.

Depression affects people in different ways and can cause a wide variety of symptoms:

Experiences range from lasting feelings of unhappiness, negativity and hopelessness, to losing interest in things that previously gave pleasure. Many people with depression also have symptoms of anxiety. Some are very tearful.

Physical symptoms include general malaise and feeling washed out and exhausted, difficulty sleeping, losing interest in food (or binge eating), reduced sex drive, and developing unidentifiable aches and pains.

Depression can be mild or severe, and many stages in between. With mild depression someone may feel out of sorts and persistently low. Severe depression can make someone feel suicidal, that life is hopeless and no longer worth living.

There are all sorts of external factors that can make someone feel depressed and most people experience some form of low mood at some time in their lives. Sometimes depression can be due to bereavement, extreme stress, a difficult home or work life, trauma, illness and a host of other reasons. Sometimes it is necessary to try and treat the root cause of the problem first, such as helping with bereavement counselling or addressing a stressful workplace. Sometimes treating the root cause will alleviate the depression on its own.

There are also some specific types of depression:

- **Seasonal affective disorder (SAD)** – depression that occurs at a particular time of year, or during a particular season.

- **Dysthymia** – continuous mild depression that lasts for two years or more. Also called persistent depressive disorder or chronic depression.

- **Prenatal depression** – depression that occurs during pregnancy. This is sometimes also called antenatal depression.

- **Postnatal depression (PND)** – depression that occurs in the first year after giving birth.

Recognising the signs someone may be depressed:

The NHS has produced a helpful self-assessment tool for people to use if they think they may be depressed https://www.nhs.uk/conditions/clinical-depression/

Further possible indicators include someone experiencing the following feelings:

- continuously low, upset or tearful

- restless, agitated or irritable

- guilty, worthless and down on yourself

- empty and numb

- isolated and unable to relate to other people

- finding no pleasure in life and no longer enjoying things that used to make you happy

- a sense of unreality and disconnect

- lack of self-confidence or self-esteem

- hopeless and despairing

- suicidal

Different behaviour changes:

- lethargy and exhaustion

- avoiding social events and activities

- self-harming or suicidal behaviour

- difficulty speaking, thinking clearly or making decisions

- difficulty remembering or concentrating

- smoking or drinking more than usual or taking drugs

- difficulty sleeping, or sleeping too much

- change in eating habits and appetite: no appetite and losing weight, or eating too much and gaining weight

- going off sick with physical aches and pains with no obvious physical cause

- changes in pace, either moving very slowly, or being restless and agitated.

Some people experience psychotic symptoms with severe depression:

It is not unusual to experience a psychotic symptom during an episode of severe depression. It does not mean someone is developing an additional mental illness.

- delusions can occur, such as paranoia

- hallucinations, such as hearing voices.

Psychotic episodes can be frightening or upsetting, so it's important to get prompt and appropriate treatment.

Treating depression

Treatment for depression can involve a combination of lifestyle changes, talking therapies and medicine.

For mild depression, depending how long it has been going on, doctors may suggest that rather than jump in with treatment, to try lifestyle changes and see if these help first. This is known as "watchful waiting". Lifestyle measures such as exercise and self-help groups have been shown to be particularly helpful.

The sort of treatment offered for depression tends to depend on the severity of symptoms.

Self-help resources

Self-help could be delivered through:

- **A self-help programme.** This may consist of a self-help manual to guide someone through specific helpful steps to help their mental health. These are usually supported by a healthcare professional, either face-to-face or over the phone.

- **A computer-based CBT programme for depression.** Many GPs can recommend computerised cognitive behavioural therapy (CCBT).

- **A physical activity programme.** GPs may recommend a group exercise class and have the ability to refer people to appropriate well-being and life-style classes. These are specifically designed for people with depression and run by qualified professionals.

Talking therapies are often used for mild or moderate depression.

There are many different talking treatments that can be effective in treating depression:

- cognitive behavioural therapy (CBT)

- group-based CBT

- interpersonal therapy (IPT)

- behavioural activation

- psychodynamic psychotherapy

- behavioural couples therapy – it can be helpful to have a long-term partner joining the therapy in order to further support the treatment.

There can be a long waiting time for talking therapies, however the Improving Access to Psychological Therapies (IAPT) programme is aiming to help people to access therapy quicker through self-referral.

Antidepressants are also sometimes prescribed.

For moderate to severe depression, a combination of talking therapy and antidepressants may be the best course of action, along with life-style changes and self-help groups. For severe depression, people may be referred to a specialist mental health team for intensive specialist talking treatments and prescribed medicine.

Medication for depression

If self-help, computerised cognitive behavioural therapy or physical activity have not helped, you might also be offered an antidepressant medication, either on its own or in combination with a talking treatment. There are different types of antidepressant:

- selective serotonin reuptake inhibitors (SSRIs)

- serotonin and norepinephrine reuptake inhibitors (SNRIs)

- tricyclics and tricyclic-related drugs

- monoamine oxidase inhibitors (MAOIs)

- other antidepressants

Different people find different medications most helpful.

Coming off medication

If someone is taking medication for depression, it's important not to stop suddenly. Withdrawal symptoms from antidepressants can be difficult to cope with and stopping suddenly can be dangerous. MIND has extremely helpful advice and help on coming off antidepressants.

NICE guidelines recommend that people continue to take antidepressants for at least six months after the conclusion of the depressive episode.

Alternative treatments

There are additional options that some people find helpful instead of, or alongside, medication and talking treatments. These include:

- arts therapies

- alternative and complementary therapies

- mindfulness

- ecotherapy

- peer support.

Helping someone who is depressed:

The CARES approach can provide a helpful structure to approaching someone you believe may be depressed:

Check for immediate life-threatening emergency. Calmly approach, reassure, assess and assist.

If they are expressing any serious self-harm or suicidal intentions, phone 999 or the Samaritans. If there is a physical first aid emergency – give immediate aid and phone 999 for an ambulance.

If you suspect an overdose – if they are unconscious and not breathing – give CPR (do not give breaths unless you have a pocket mask to protect you from whatever they have ingested)

If they are unconscious and breathing – put them into the recovery position, keep checking for breathing and phone for an ambulance.

If they are conscious, encourage them to stay still, so as not to increase their metabolism. Try and establish what they have taken and how much. Do not give them anything to eat or drink, or try and make them sick. Monitor them closely and phone for an ambulance.

Do not drive them to the hospital as they could deteriorate or lose consciousness whilst in transit. Better to call for an ambulance to give immediate aid and monitor them closely whilst on the way to the hospital.

Do not leave them alone.

If there is no obvious life-threatening emergency, calmly approach, reassure, assess and assist.

Actively listen without judgment

Recommend sources of immediate help – identify if there are any obvious sources of stress that you might be able to assist with.

Encourage to seek professional help

Suggest possible self-help and other support options for better mental health

There is a wealth of resources in our section at the back of the book.

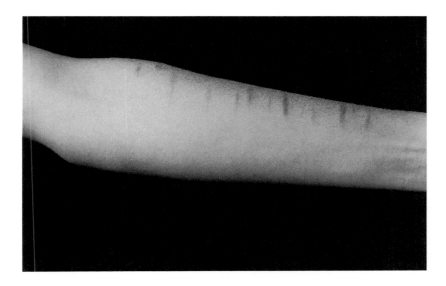

Self-harm

Self-harm occurs when someone hurts themselves as a way of dealing with overwhelming feelings, painful memories or experiences.

People that self-harm may feel a short-term sense of release, but the cause of distress will not have gone away.

What is self-harm?

Self-harm is when you hurt yourself on purpose. You usually do it because something else feels wrong. It seems like the only way to let those feelings out.

Self-harm is when you hurt yourself as a way of dealing with very difficult feelings, painful memories or overwhelming situations and experiences

How someone might self-harm themselves:

- Cutting, scratching, or burning their skin

- Head banging

- Punching, slapping, pinching, or hitting themselves

- Continually picking at scabs

- Misusing alcohol, drugs or overdosing

- Starving themselves, making themselves sick or using laxatives

- Excessively exercising

- Pulling their hair out

- Poisoning themselves with medication or chemicals

Signs someone may be self-harming:

- Unexplained cuts, bruises, marks like cigarette burns on wrists, arms, thighs, chest or stomach

- Covering up at all times – even in hot weather

- Signs of low self-esteem, continually putting themselves down

- Possible signs of depression, lack of motivation, tearfulness, disinterest

- Avoidance of social events and social contact, withdrawn

- Seem to have frequent 'accidents'

How common is self harm:

Self-harming is a very common behaviour in young people. It affects around one in 12 people, with 10% of 15-16 year olds self-harming.

However there has recently been an alarming rise in younger children aged from 9-12 self-harming to the extent that they require admission to hospital. This has resulted in about 10 children a week being seen in A&E.

Self-injury admissions for girls in this age group is twice as high as for boys.

There has also been an increase in the rate of admissions for 13 to 17-year-olds, which has doubled in seven years. 12 young people per day are seen in hospital because of self-harm.

However, the majority of children and young people who self-harm do not need hospital treatment.

People that self-harm, usually do so because of another problem. It can become a distraction and way of coping when they feel they don't have any other way of dealing with these issues.

Sometimes people don't understand why they self-harm and find themselves unable to stop.

Sometimes someone may try to seriously hurt themselves in order to commit suicide; this usually has a different motivation. Most people who self-harm do not suicidal intentions.

Get help early: If you think you are self-harming, talk to someone - a parent or relative you trust, perhaps a teacher, family member or youth worker or your GP.

Why talk to your GP?

Self-harm can be a sign of other disorders that you need help with - such as depression or anxiety - and they can refer you to the right people for treatment. You may also be referred to Child and Adolescent Mental Health Services (CAMHS) so you can have an assessment of the right treatment for you.

Treating Injuries

Your injuries should be treated with prompt and appropriate first aid.

How to help someone who you think may be self-harming:

Self-harm encompasses a wide range of things people deliberately do to themselves to cause physical pain or damage.

It is most common for people to cut the arms or the back of the legs. However it could involve burning, biting, hitting oneself, banging their head, pulling out their hair (trichotilliomania), inserting objects into the body or taking overdoses.

Reasons for self-harm

Sometimes there is no specific reason for someone to self-harm, it appears to generate a release from overwhelming negative or disturbing feelings. Sometimes they may self-harm to help cope with negative feelings and difficult experiences, to feel more in control, or to punish themselves.

When speaking with someone who is self-harming they may explain they do it to:

- reduce tension

- induce physical pain to distract from emotional pain

- help express emotions such as hurt, anger or frustration

- regain control over feelings or problems

- punish themselves or others

It may start due to anxiety, depression, low self-esteem, poor body image, gender identity, sexuality, abuse, school problems, bullying, social media pressure, family or friendship troubles and bereavement or a myriad of other issues.

Self-harming can become a habit that is hard to stop.

How to help if you suspect someone is self-harming:

Keep an eye open for the following signs:

- unexplained cuts, burns, bite-marks, bruises or bald patches

- they are fastidious about covering up; avoiding swimming, short sleeved tops of shorts or changing in the presence of others. (although this can be a normal part of growing up too)

- finding bloody tissues in waste bins

- becoming withdrawn or isolated from friends and family

- low mood, lack of interest in life, depression or outbursts of anger

- blaming themselves for problems or expressing feelings of failure, uselessness, hopelessness or worthlessness.

How to open the conversation:

If you are helping someone who is self-harming, the same CARES method will help.

Check for any immediate life-threatening injuries and if so, ask their permission to treat: e.g. treat bleeding by applying firm pressure. Ensure you are safe and remove the danger that has caused their injuries.

Approach non-judgementally, allow them to talk and actively listen with compassion. Offer immediate support and encourage them to seek further help.

Remain calm, do not ignore their injuries, or overly focus on them. Speak to them as a whole person without focussing on their injuries or actions.

Ensure they know you care about them and are doing your best to help.

Listen to what they say and help them to be in control of their decisions.

See if there is a close friend or family member that they are happy to talk to and help them contact them if they would like to.

Their GP should be the best professional person for them to see. They should then work with them to establish if there is an underlying reason for their self-harm.

It can be an incredibly difficult conversation for parents, teachers, friends, family and trusted adults to broach:

It is more important than ever not to appear judgemental.

1. Avoid interrogating and asking lots of questions all at once.

2. Keep an eye on them but avoid 'policing' them because this can increase their risk of self-harming. It is something they are likely to do in private.

3. Remember the self-harm is a coping mechanism. It is a symptom of an underlying problem.

4. Keep all lines of communication open, it may not be the right time or place. You might not be the right person for them to speak to. Tell them it is okay for them to speak to someone else and encourage them to get help. They may feel ashamed of their self-harm and find it very difficult to talk about.

5. Try not to be angry or disappointed with what they are doing.

6. Keep firm boundaries and a sense of normality, this will help the child feel secure and emotionally stable.

7. If you feel confident, you can ask them whether removing whatever they are using to self-harm is likely to cause them to use something less sanitary to self-harm with, or whether it reduces temptation. This can be a difficult question to ask and if you are not confident to ask this seek professional advice.

8. Seek professional help. They are likely to need a risk assessment from a qualified mental health professional. Their GP may be able to refer them to the local Child and Adolescent Mental Health Services (CAMHS).

9. Discovering and responding to self-harm can be a traumatic experience for someone who cares about the child who is self-harming. Many people feel guilt, shame, anger, sadness, frustration and despair – but it's not your fault.

Please visit the resource section at the back of this book for specific help for self-harm.

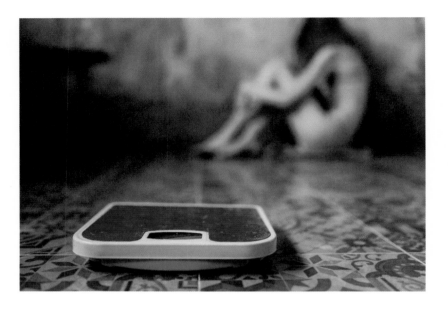

Eating Disorders

An eating disorder occurs when someone develops an unhealthy attitude towards food which can take over their everyday life and make them ill.

Food plays an integral part in our lives and we all spend time thinking about what we have eaten, or what we are going to eat. Sometimes we may try to eat more healthily, try a diet, have cravings, eat more than usual or lose our appetite. Changing your eating habits every now and again is normal.

Sometimes food and eating becomes an obsession and it feels like it's an overwhelming part of life. This is when it becomes a problem.

When someone has an eating disorder, they will often eat too much or too little, or binge and make themselves sick, or use laxatives. They can become obsessed with their body weight and appearance and what they see when they look in the mirror can be very different to the reality.

It is often believed that if someone has an eating problem they will always noticeably appear under or overweight – this is not the case! Anyone, regardless of their weight, age or gender can be seriously affected by an eating disorder.

People can develop eating problems which can sometime go on to become an eating disorder.

- An eating disorder is a medical diagnosis based on eating patterns, medical tests, weight, blood and body mass index (BMI).

- An eating problem is a difficult relationship with food. This can be just as hard to live with as a diagnosed eating disorder.

Eating problems tend not to be just about food. They can be a way of coping with difficult things and painful feelings, which the person may find hard to express, face or resolve. Focusing on food can be a way of disguising these problems, sometimes the individual themselves may not realise this is the case.

Lots of people have different eating habits. You might be known as a fussy eater, eat loads one day, less another day, try diets and want to eat more or less healthily. But none of these mean you have an eating problem.

However, if you focus on controlling what or how much you eat, or if you have urges to eat and then make yourself sick (bulimia), or try using laxatives afterwards, these are signs you could have a problem.

Eating problems are common and they affect people with any body shape or lifestyle.

How common are eating disorders?

Between 1.25 and 3.4 million people in the UK are affected by an eating disorder. Around 25% of those affected by an eating disorder are male. Most eating disorders develop during adolescence, although there are cases of eating disorders developing in children as young as 6 and in adults in their 70's.

All kinds of things can lead to eating problems or disorders. Sometimes people develop an eating problem to try and control something in their life when they are feeling worried, stressed or feeling out of control. Sometimes social media and media portrayal can lead people to feel they have to look a certain way, or be a certain weight which may not be healthy.

Often what someone sees when they look in the mirror is totally different to what they really look like.

Signs someone could have an eating problem

Here are some indicators that someone could be experiencing an eating problem:

If they are regularly:

- Not wanting to eat

- eating when not hungry

- obsessing about their body (e.g. being too fat, need a 6 pack or more muscles)

- eating only certain types of things or following fad diets

- being afraid of gaining weight

- their appearance may change, becoming noticeably fatter or thinner

- making themselves sick

- may eat very slowly and cut their food up very small or eat a lot of food very fast

- no longer enjoying eating socially or leaving the table quickly (to be sick or hide food or visit the bathroom)

- obsessing about buying or cooking food for others

- being secretive about eating and preoccupied with food

- being self-conscious about eating in front of others

- struggling to concentrate and feeling tired a lot

- becoming depressed and anxious

- appearing unwell and sluggish

- losing their spontaneity and no longer wanting to travel or to go anywhere new

- frequently comparing their body weight or image with others.

Many people manage to hide their eating problems – sometimes they can successfully manage this for a very long time.

A person's weight on its own does not determine whether they have a problem.

Being able to control how much they eat often gives a feeling of order but can lead to more serious issues.

Some eating problems become serious mental health conditions that need professional intervention to diagnose and treat.

In serious cases and without the right kind of support and treatment, they can even result in death, which is why it is so important to get help as soon as possible.

Recovering from an eating disorder can be a long process, but with the right help a full recovery is possible.

What to do if you think you have an eating problem

Speak to your GP for advice. Sometimes learning to eat normally again can be hard work, so your doctor can help you get the support you need. They might suggest talking therapies that involve the whole family. They will help you deal with the issues that may have triggered the eating problem.

The doctor may also want to measure your weight to assess your BMI (Body Mass Index) –many people are nervous about this; however it is vital to remember that they don't want to judge, they need this information to help.

Avoid apps, accounts or websites that contribute to your negative body image and your relationship with eating.

Eating problems and links with other mental health problems

Often people with eating problems also have other mental health problems, such as depression, anxiety or obsessive-compulsive disorders. An anxiety disorder called body dysmorphic disorder results in extreme anxiety around body image and often leads to eating disorders.

For some people, eating problems are linked to self-harm – and this may lead them to hurt themselves in other ways too. Sometimes someone can develop a phobia around certain foods, that can become overwhelming and lead to eating problems and for others it could be related to self-esteem. Some people don't know how or why it has happened and do not realise they have a problem.

135

Check for life-threatening problems. Calmly approach, reassure, assess & assist.

Before approaching the person, it is helpful to take time to familiarise yourself with the symptoms and treatments of eating disorders so you are have a greater understanding about what you suspect they might be experiencing. This will help you approach more sensitively and with greater empathy.

Choose an appropriate, safe, comfortable space where you are unlikely to be disturbed.

Don't approach them to talk about this at mealtimes, in an eating environment, or when other people are around.

Actively listen without judgment

Ask open questions and explain why you are worried in an open and honest manner. Ask how they are feeling and if you can help?

Try not to focus on food or bodyweight.

Incredibly important to listen openly and without judgement.

Recommend sources of immediate help – be particularly aware of signs of crisis

See if there is anything practical you can do to alleviate some of their immediate stress?

Encourage to seek professional help

Explain that you think their symptoms indicate a need to seek professional help

The person may react positively to having a helping hand and feel a sense of relief that someone has noticed there is a problem.

Alternatively (and more likely), the person may deny there is a problem and be reluctant to seek professional help.

Try not to reason with them, or be angry if your help is dismissed, let them know you will be there for them if they need you.

Reassure the person that they can be helped and with the right support, could feel a lot better.

If they feel comfortable getting help, the best person for them to see in the first instance is their GP. Ideally they would visit their GP with a close friend or relative.

There are a variety of online self-help therapies that GPs can refer to, that many people find helpful.

In addition, GPs can refer someone to talking treatments such as CBT and help the person to access support networks.

- **Cognitive behavioural therapy for eating disorders (CBT-ED)**. This is an adapted form of CBT specifically for treatment of eating disorders, including anorexia. There are alternative forms of CBT for bulimia nervosa (CBT-BN) and binge eating disorder (CBT-BED).

- For anorexia, someone should be offered up to 40 sessions, with twice weekly sessions in the first two or three weeks.

- For bulimia someone should be offered at least 20 sessions, and may be offered twice weekly sessions at first.

- For binge eating disorder someone should be offered group CBT sessions at first.

- **Family therapy.** This means working through issues as a family with the support of a therapist and exploring family dynamics or situations that might have prompted the feelings underlying an eating disorder. It can be extremely helpful for the whole family to understand the best way to support and help them recover.

Suggest possible self-help and other support options for better mental health

For useful resources for Eating Disorders, please visits the Resource section at the back of this book

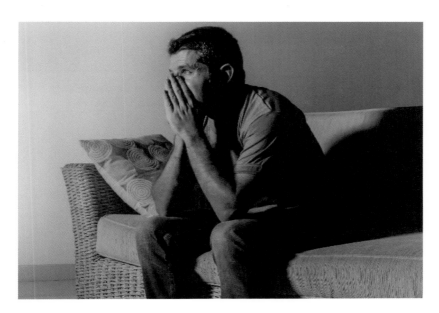

Suicide

Suicide is the act of intentionally taking one's own life.

Suicidal feelings can involve having abstract thoughts about ending your life or feeling that people would be better off without you. Or it can mean thinking about methods of suicide or making clear plans to take your own life.

When someone is feeling suicidal, they might be scared or confused by these feelings and may find the feelings overwhelming.

However, feeling suicidal is sadly not uncommon and many people think about suicide at some point in their lifetime.

What does it feel like to be suicidal?

Different people have different experiences of suicidal feelings. Some people are overwhelmed and unable to cope with the feeling. Sometimes is it more a realisation that they cannot go on living life as it stands.

- Sometimes people who are suicidal feel:

- hopeless, like there is no point in living

- tearful and overwhelmed by negative thoughts

- unbearable, continual pain

- useless, not wanted or not needed by others

- desperate, without any other options

- like everyone would be better off without them

- remote, physically numb or cut off from reality

- fascinated by death.

What indicators might there be:

As part of their depression and suicidal thoughts you might notice the following:

- they look tired, weary and exhausted

- a change in appetite, weight gain or loss

- they may appear unkempt, or have a change in appearance, not bothering with hair, makeup or clothes as they would have previously.

- appear to avoid being with other people

- making a will or give away possessions

- struggle to communicate

- express self-loathing and low self-esteem.

The type of suicidal feelings people have, varies person to person, in particular in terms of:

- **how intense they are** – suicidal feelings are more overwhelming for some people than others. They can build up gradually or be intense from the start. They can be more or less severe at different times and may change quickly.

- **how long they last** – suicidal feelings are sometimes fleeting and disappear on their own but might still be very intense. They may come and go or last for a long time.

Many people find it very hard to talk about suicidal feelings – this can be because they are worried about how others will react or because they cannot find the words. They might hide how they are feeling and try to convince friends or family that they are coping.

The Samaritans website also has a helpful page for anyone worried that someone they know is feeling suicidal. This page includes a list of warning signs that you may notice, although there might not be any signs or you might not be able to tell. Correctly interpreting how someone else is feeling can be difficult so it's very important not to blame yourself if you aren't able to spot the signs that someone is feeling suicidal.

Who is at risk of suicide?

Anyone can have suicidal feelings, whatever their background or situation in life. Suicidal feelings have a wide range of possible causes. Suicidal feelings can be a symptom of an existing mental health problem or episode of mental distress, or sometimes a side effect of medication – bizarrely many antidepressants can cause suicidal thoughts. If someone is feeling suicidal it is important to be aware of medication they are taking, which could be causing or aggravating these feelings. However, no medication should be stopped without medical advice and guidance.

If someone feels suicidal, they often find their feelings may become more intense when they:

- drink alcohol

- use street drugs

- have sleep problems

Some groups have been shown to more at risk of suicide:

Statistically LGBTQ people are more likely to take their own lives. People can also be more vulnerable to suicide if:

- **they have attempted suicide before** – if someone has previously tried to end their life, there is a greater than average chance they may try to do so again in future

- **they have self-harmed in the past** – self-harm isn›t the same as feeling suicidal, but statistics show that someone who has self-harmed is likely to be more at risk of suicide

- **they have lost someone to suicide** – family members of someone who has committed suicide are also more at risk of taking their own lives

If someone is experiencing an immediate crisis, get emergency aid.

Whilst waiting for the emergency services, MIND has some really helpful resources to assist the person to get through the next few minutes.

What to do if the person is in a life-threatening condition:

If they are unconscious and not breathing – commence CPR. Protect yourself if giving breaths.

If they are bleeding, apply direct pressure to the wound.

If they are unconscious and breathing, put into the recovery position and keep checking for breathing.

Phone for an ambulance.

CARES – Approaching someone you suspect may have suicidal feelings

Check for life-threatening problems. Calmly approach, reassure, assess & assist.

Actively listen without judgment

Recommend sources of immediate help – be particularly aware of signs of crisis

Encourage to seek professional help

Suggest possible self-help and other support options for better mental health

> There is a wealth of support for people experiencing suicidal thoughts – please see our Resources section at the back of the book.

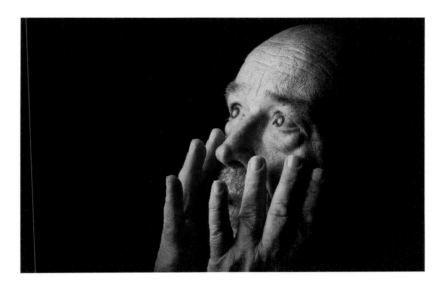

Psychosis:

Psychosis is a general term used when someone loses touch with commonly accepted reality. They experience a mental health issue that changes the way they think, perceive and behave, which can seriously disrupt their life.

The most common types of psychotic experiences are hallucinations, delusions and disorganised thinking and speech.

The most common psychotic disorders are:

- severe depression

- schizophrenia

- bipolar disorder

- schizoaffective disorder

- paranoid personality disorder or schizotypal personality disorder

- postpartum psychosis

- delusional disorder

- psychotic depression

- drug induced psychosis

It is most common for psychosis to develop in adolescence.

What causes psychosis?

The cause of psychosis can be different for everyone, and research into it is happening all the time. Psychosis could be triggered by a number of things; some examples of these are:

Physical illness or injury can cause someone to hallucinate. An infection, extremely high fever, head injury, lead or mercury poisoning can lead someone to see things that aren't there. Some people with Alzheimer's disease or Parkinson's disease may also experience hallucinations or delusions.

Abuse or trauma may also make it more likely that someone will experience psychosis.

For people who have already experienced psychosis, using recreational drugs can make the symptoms worse, in particular, high-potency cannabis ('skunk').

Alcohol and smoking. Drinking alcohol and smoking may stop medication from effectively treating symptoms, making relapse more likely.

Prescribed medication. psychosis can occur as a side effect of some prescribed drugs or when coming off psychiatric drugs.

Some people find that if they are susceptible to psychotic episodes, they can be triggered by

- life events

- changes in mood or hormones

- a different diet

- lack of sleep

Early signs of possible psychosis:

- Changes in emotion and motivation

- Depression, anxiety and irritability

- Suspiciousness

- Inappropriate reaction to emotion

- Changes in appetite

- Reduced energy and motivation

Changes in thinking and perception:

- Strange ideas

- Difficulty with concentration or attention

- Sense that they or other people have altered in some way, or are acting differently

- Changes in perception, seeing hearing or smelling things with greater (or lesser) intensity

Changes in behaviour

- Social isolation or withdrawal

- Struggling to carry out work or join social outings

- Sleep disturbance

Stress and relaxation techniques can help some people control the severity or number of episodes they experience. Physical exercise, being outdoors and a good diet can also be helpful. If someone has a predisposition to psychosis they are strongly advised to avoid drugs and alcohol.

If early signs of psychosis are acted upon and promptly treated, there is a far greater chance of someone making a full recovery.

CARES approach to Psychosis:

Psychosis can be frightening, both for the people experiencing it, and for those trying to help them.

Psychosis

- affects someone's behaviour and can disrupt their life

- can make them feel very tired or overwhelmed

- often makes them feel anxious, scared, threatened or confused

- may leave them finding it difficult to trust some organisations or people.

It is particularly important to approach someone experiencing a psychotic episode cautiously and sensitively. Remember that what they are experiencing is very real to them and it is frustrating and upsetting if they feel someone doesn't believe them.

If someone is having an acute psychotic episode, you may not be the best person to approach them. If they are not in touch with reality, you could unwittingly make things worse. Therefore, it may be more appropriate to stand back, ensure they are safe, but call for the emergency services professionals to come and help.

If someone is experiencing an immediate crisis, get emergency aid.

If the person is behaving aggressively:

- Stay back and observe from a safe distance. Ensure you have a safe exit, should you need to leave.

- Call the police, if you think this is the most appropriate course of action. Ask them to send a plain clothes officer if possible. If you have phoned for an ambulance as well, they may not attend until the police are there to help. Involving the police may exacerbate the situation, particularly if the person is feeling paranoid. However, if they are a danger to themselves, or someone else, then this is the best course of action.

- If you are speaking with the person, remain calm, talk slowly, quietly and simply. Turn your phone to silent so it won't suddenly ring, turn off the radio or TV and try to reduce additional noise and distractions.

- Keep at a distance; avoid prolonged, direct eye contact. Don't touch the person and respect their space.

- Don't try to reason with them.

- Empathise with their distress, but don't pretend to experience their hallucinations or delusions.

- Comply with reasonable requests as this will help them feel a sense of control. However, do not make promises that you can't keep.

Check for life-threatening problems. **If safe and appropriate (see above) - C**almly approach, reassure, assess & assist.

Actively listen without judgment

Recommend sources of immediate help – be particularly aware of signs of crisis – if they are delusional and experiencing a psychotic episode, then ensure their safety and the safety of those they are responsible for.

Help ensure care arrangements are in place for any people or pets they may have responsibility for.

Assist with immediate practical solutions that are within your control.

Contact next of kin or a close family friend if they would like you to and if appropriate.

Encourage to seek professional help – if they are in a psychotic state, they will need emergency professional help **now**.

If they are calmly talking to you about psychotic episodes that they experience from time to time, then this is a good point to signpost them to different options.

When someone experiences a psychotic episode for the first time, they will be referred to an 'early intervention team'. This Mental Health Team will make a detailed assessment of their needs and work out the most appropriate treatment plan.

People with complex needs will be supported by a 'care programme approach' which consists of four stages:

- **Assessment** – the person's condition will be formally assessed

- **Care plan** – a care plan will be created based on the outcome of the assessment

- **Key worker** – a professional will be appointed as the first point of contact

- **Review** – the person's treatment plan will be reviewed and followed up at regular intervals

Suggest possible self-help and other support options for better mental health – as above. This is only appropriate when they are not experiencing psychosis.

> **For helpful support for Psychosis, please see our Resources section at the back of this book.**

Understanding personality disorders:

Our personality is the unique amalgamation of our thoughts, feelings and behaviour. It identifies who we are and although we may modify it for certain social circumstances and interactions, it remains fairly constant throughout our lives.

Someone with a personality disorder often behaves differently in social situations. They may relate to others in an unusual way and their interaction in terms of thoughts, feelings, perceptions and behaviours may be different as a result.

Currently psychiatrists generally use a diagnostic system which identifies ten types of personality disorder. These are grouped into three categories.

Suspicious:

- Paranoid personality disorder

- Schizoid personality disorder

- Schizotypal personality disorder

- Antisocial personality disorder

Emotional and impulsive:

- Borderline personality disorder (BPD)

- Histrionic personality disorder

- Narcissistic personality disorder

Anxious:

- Avoidant personality disorder

- Dependent personality disorder

- Obsessive compulsive personality disorder (OCPD)

Many people with personality disorders develop other mental health problems such as depression, anxiety or substance misuse.

Sometimes their condition may lead them to experience periods of psychosis.

As a Mental Health First Aider you are not diagnosing anyone. You are recognising signs that someone may be struggling with their mental health and offering help and support.

For people with a personality disorder, it is necessary to have additional empathy and understanding to ensure that you approach them in a particularly sensitive manner.

It is most likely that you will be helping them obtain help for an exacerbation of issues such as depression, anxiety or psychosis.

If the person already has a diagnosis and is experiencing a crisis, then they are likely to be under the care of the Mental Health Team and have an emergency support number to call in just such a situation.

Understanding Bi-Polar Disorder:

Bipolar disorder is a mental health problem that predominantly affects your mood. People with bipolar disorder, often experience episodes where they feel:

- **manic or hypomanic episodes** (feeling high)

- **depressive episodes** (feeling low)

- **potentially some psychotic symptoms** during manic or depressed episodes

Everyone has variations in their mood, but in bipolar disorder these changes can be extreme and have a major effect on their day to day life.

The exact cause of bipolar disorder is unknown, but some people may be more susceptible to develop the condition, due possibly to genetics or a chemical imbalance of neurotransmitters in the brain. Childhood trauma and stressful life events may also prompt someone to develop bi-polar disorder.

About manic episodes

Mania can come on without warning and last for in excess of a week at a time. It severely impacts upon someone's ability to cope with day to day life. Severe mania is very serious and people frequently need to be treated in hospital.

During a manic episode:

Someone might be:

- ecstatically happy, euphoric or with a profound sense of wellbeing

- uncontrollably excited, unable to get words out fast enough

- irritable and agitated

- overly friendly with an increased sexual appetite

- behaving inappropriately, without inhibitions

- easily distracted, racing thoughts, totally unable to concentrate

- over-confident, risk taking and adventurous, with a sense of invincibility

- acting like they have superpowers

- spending money like water

- misusing drugs and alcohol

- existing with very little sleep

About hypomanic episodes

Hypomania is similar to mania, but at a more manageable level.

It usually lasts for a shorter time

It isn't accompanied by psychosis

Following a manic or hypomanic episode the person might:

- feel very unhappy or ashamed about how they behaved, or have no memory of the period at all

- have taken on responsibilities that now feel unmanageable

- feel very tired and need a lot of sleep and rest

About depressive episodes

During a depressive episode someone might be:

- down, upset or tearful

- tired or sluggish

- unable to enjoy things that used to give them pleasure

- have lost their confidence or sense of worth

- agitated and tense

- tired as they have difficulty sleeping or waking

- misusing drugs or alcohol

- self-harming or suicidal

- eating too little or too much

Many people find that a depressive episode can feel harder to deal with than manic or hypomanic episodes. The contrast between high and low moods may make the depression seem even deeper.

About mixed episodes

Mixed episodes (also called 'mixed states') are when someone experiences symptoms of depression and mania or hypomania simultaneously or quickly one after the other. This can be particularly difficult to cope with, as:

- it is confusing for them to work out what they are feeling and what help they need

- it is an exhausting mix of extreme emotions

- they may be more likely to act on suicidal thoughts and feelings – **really important for a mental health first aider to understand this might be the case.**

Psychotic symptoms associated with bi-polar disorder can include:

- delusions, such as paranoia

- hallucinations, such as hearing voices

Not everyone with a diagnosis of bipolar disorder experiences psychosis, but some people do. It's more common during manic episodes but can happen during depressive episodes too.

Someone with a diagnosis of bi-polar disorder should be under the care of the Mental Health Team. They should ideally be contacted in the first instance and there should be an emergency number readily available.

As a Mental Health First Aider, when approaching someone experiencing a bi-polar crisis, adhere to the CARES approach:

Ensure your safety, their safety and that of those around them.

Be ready to help with whatever they need.

If you are not the best person to help them, contact a close friend or family member and the emergency services if necessary.

Understanding Schizophrenia:

Schizophrenia is a long-term mental health disorder that affects how we think, feel and behave. Schizophrenia causes a range of different psychological symptoms and can make life very difficult to cope with.

Contrary to popular opinion, schizophrenics do not have a split personality, nor do they tend to be violent. However, they may experience extreme psychotic symptoms that can leave them delusional, hallucinating, or out of touch with reality.

Someone experiencing a relapse of their schizophrenia could experience:

- hallucinations, such as hearing voices or seeing things others don't

- delusions (which could include paranoid delusions) – strong beliefs that others don't share

- disorganised thinking and speech

- a dishevelled appearance and lack of interest in things around them

- difficulty concentrating

- a need to avoid people

- a sense of disconnect, not engaged in life around them

- suspiciousness, confusion or distrust of other people or particular groups, like strangers or people in authority

If helping someone experiencing an exacerbation of their symptoms, they should be under the care of the Mental Health Team. Contact a close friend or family member and the Mental Health Team in the first instance.

Follow the CARES approach, whilst ensuring your own safety, their safety and the safety of anyone around them, particularly if they have been taking drugs or alcohol.

USEFUL RESOURCES and REFERENCE SECTION:

Useful resources for drug and alcohol misuse

Talk to Frank is an incredibly helpful information source for drug advise:

https://www.talktofrank.com/get-help/find-support-near-you

https://www.nhs.uk/live-well/healthy-body/drug-addiction-getting-help/

https://www.mind.org.uk/information-support/guides-to-support-and-services/addiction-and-dependency/addiction-and-dependency-resources/

NHS Live Well
nhs.uk/livewell
Advice, tips and tools to help with health and wellbeing.

Beating Addictions
beatingaddictions.co.uk
Information about a range of addictive behaviours and treatments.

Sources of support

Addaction
addaction.org.uk
Supports people with drug, alcohol or mental health problems, and their friends and family.

Adfam
adfam.org.uk
Information and support for friends and family of people with drug or alcohol problems.
Alcoholics Anonymous (AA)
0800 9177 650
alcoholics-anonymous.org.uk
Help and support for anyone with alcohol problems.

The Alliance
m-alliance.org
User-led organisation that provides information and advocacy for people accessing treatment for drug and alcohol problems.

Drink aware

https://www.drinkaware.co.uk/

Drugwise – giving evidence-based information on drugs, alcohol and tobacco

https://www.drugwise.org.uk/

FRANK

0300 123 6600
talktofrank.com
Confidential advice and information about drugs, their effects and the law.

National Association for Children of Alcoholics

0800 358 3456
nacoa.org.uk
Provides information, advice and support for everyone affected by a parent's drinking, including adults.

Narcotics Anonymous

0300 999 1212
ukna.org
Support for anyone who wants to stop using drugs.

Release

020 7324 2989
release.org.uk
National charity that gives free and confidential advice about drugs and the law.

Turning Point

turning-point.co.uk

Provides health and social care services for people with drug, alcohol and mental health problems.

Useful contacts for anxiety

Anxiety Care UK

anxietycare.org.uk

Helps people with anxiety disorders.

Anxiety UK

03444 775 774 (helpline)

07537 416 905 (text)

anxietyuk.org.uk

Advice and support for people living with anxiety.

British Association for Counselling and Psychotherapy (BACP)

bacp.co.uk

Professional body for talking therapy and counselling. Provides information and a list of accredited therapists.

Improving Access to Psychological Therapies (IAPT)

nhs.uk/service-search/find-a-psychological-therapies-service

Information about local NHS therapy and counselling services, which you can often self-refer to (England only).

National Institute for Health and Care Excellence (NICE)

nice.org.uk

Produces guidelines on best practice in healthcare.

NHS Service Finder

nhs.uk/service-search

Searchable database of NHS services in England.

No More Panic

nomorepanic.co.uk

Provides information, support and advice for those with panic disorder, anxiety, phobias or OCD, including a forum and chat room.

No Panic

0844 967 4848

nopanic.org.uk

Provides a helpline, step-by-step programmes, and support for people with anxiety disorders.

Samaritans

116 123 (freephone)

jo@samaritans.org

Freepost RSRB-KKBY-CYJK

PO Box 90 90

Stirling FK8 2SA

samaritans.org

Open 24/7 for anyone who needs to talk. You can visit some branches in person. They also have a Welsh Language Line on 0300 123 3011 (7pm–11pm every day).

Triumph Over Phobia (TOP UK)

topuk.org
Provides self-help therapy groups and support for those with OCD, phobias and related anxiety disorders.

Helpful advice and support for PTSD

Assist Trauma Care is a charity that specialises in PTSD

http://assisttraumacare.org.uk/

Combat Stress – combatstress.org.uk

Treatment and support for British Armed Forces Veterans

Rape Crisis – rapecrisis.org.uk

Disaster Action – disasteraction.org.uk

Information and support for people affected by major disasters.

Victim Support – victimsupport.org.uk

Providing support and information for victims and witnesses of crime

Useful resources for Depression

Mind's services

- Helplines – our Infoline provide information and support by phone, email, and text.

- Local Minds – provide face-to-face services, such as talking therapies, peer support and advocacy, across England and Wales.

- Elefriends – our supportive online community for anyone experiencing a mental health problem.

Other organisations

Anxiety UK

03444 775 774 (helpline)
07537 416 905 (text)
anxietyuk.org.uk
Advice and support for people living with anxiety.

Big White Wall

bigwhitewall.com
Online mental health community. Free in some areas through your GP, employer or university.

British Association for Counselling and Psychotherapy (BACP)

bacp.co.uk
Professional body for talking therapy and counselling. Provides information and a list of accredited therapists.

Campaign Against Living Miserably (CALM)

0800 58 58 58 (UK helpline)

0808 802 58 58 (London helpline)

thecalmzone.net

Provides listening services, information and support for men at risk of suicide, including a web chat.

Cruse Bereavement Care

0808 808 1677

cruse.org.uk

Information and support after a bereavement.

Depression UK

depressionuk.org

Depression self-help organisation made up of individuals and local groups.

Do-it

do-it.org

Lists UK volunteering opportunities.

The National Association for People Abused in Childhood (NAPAC)

0808 801 0331

napac.org.uk

A charity supporting adult survivors of any form of childhood abuse. Provides a support line and local support services.

National Institute for Health and Care Excellence (NICE)

nice.org.uk

Produces guidelines on best practice in healthcare.

NCT

0300 330 0700

nct.org.uk

Provides information, support and classes for parents.

NHS UK

nhs.uk

Information about health problems and treatments, including details of local NHS services in England.

Maytree Trust

maytree.org.uk

A helpline for people experiencing suicidal feelings

Papyrus HOPELINEUK

0800 068 41 41

07786 209697 (text)

papyrus-uk.org

Confidential support for under-35s at risk of suicide and others who are concerned about them.

Samaritans

116-123

samaritans.org

Freepost RSRB-KKBY-CYJK

PO Box 90 90

Stirling FK8 2SA

jo@samaritans.org

24-hour emotional support for anyone who needs to talk.

Sane

0300 304 7000

sane.org.uk

Offers emotional support and information for anyone affected by mental health problems.

UK Council for Psychotherapy (UKCP)

psychotherapy.org.uk

Professional body for the education, training and accreditation of psychotherapists and psychotherapeutic counsellors. Provides online register of psychotherapists offering different talking treatments privately.

Organisations that can help with Self-harm

Self harm

- Mind – call 0300 123 3393 or text 86463 (9am to 6pm on weekdays)

- Harmless – email info@harmless.org.uk harmless.org. uk Provides a range of services for people who self-harm along with support for their friends and families.

- <u>Self-injury Support</u> (for women and girls)

- <u>CALM</u> (for men)

- <u>Young Minds Parents Helpline</u> – call <u>0808 802 5544</u> (9.30am to 4pm on weekdays) youngminds.org.uk Advice and support for anyone worried about someone under 25.

- <u>National Self Harm Network forums</u> nshn.co.uk Well monitored self-harm support forum

If you struggle with suicidal thoughts or are supporting someone else, the <u>Staying Safe website</u> provides information on how to make a safety plan. It includes video tutorials and online templates to guide you through the process.

Free <u>distrACT app</u>. quick and discreet access to information and advice about self-harm and suicidal thoughts.

<u>Alumina</u> – free online help for people self-harming <u>https://www.selfharm.co.uk/</u> - free online self-harm support for 14-19s

Lifesigns – lifesigns.org.uk Guidance and support network from people who understand.

Young Minds Parents helpline – youngminds.org.uk Advice and support for anyone worried about someone under 25.

NHS Choices – wealth of information on many topics

Mind – a great resource website

Useful resources for Eating Disorders:

Anorexia and Bulimia Care (ABC)

03000 11 12 13

anorexiabulimiacare.org.uk

Advice and support for anyone affected by eating problems.

Association for Family Therapy and Systemic Practice

aft.org.uk

Information about family therapy, including a directory of therapists.

B-EAT

b-eat.co.uk

Beat is the UK's leading charity supporting anyone affected by eating disorders.

0808 801 0711 (youthline)

0808 801 0811 (studentline)

beateatingdisorders.co.uk

Under 18s helpline, webchat and online support groups for people with eating disorders, such as anorexia and bulimia.

British Association for Behavioural and Cognitive Psychotherapies (BABCP)

babcp.com

Information about cognitive behavioural therapy and related treatments, including details of accredited therapists.

British Association for Counselling and Psychotherapy (BACP)

bacp.co.uk

Professional body for talking therapy and counselling. Provides information and a list of accredited therapists.

Men Get Eating Disorders Too

mengetedstoo.co.uk

Support and advice for men with eating disorders

National Centre for Eating Disorders

eating-disorders.org.uk

Everything you need to know about eating disorder treatments, information and professional training.

NICE

nice.org.uk

Produces guidelines on best practice in healthcare.

Overeaters Anonymous Great Britain

oagb.org.uk

Local support groups for people with eating problems.

Papyrus HOPELINEUK

0800 068 41 41

07786 209697 (text)

papyrus-uk.org

Confidential support for under-35s at risk of suicide and others who are concerned about them.

Samaritans

116 123 (freephone)

jo@samaritans.org

Freepost RSRB-KKBY-CYJK

PO Box 90 90

Stirling FK8 2SA

samaritans.org

Open 24/7 for anyone who needs to talk. You can visit some branches in person. They also have a Welsh Language Line on 0300 123 3011 (7pm–11pm every day).

SEED

seedeatingdisorders.org.uk

A group of ordinary people with first-hand experience of eating disorders.

Student Minds

studentminds.org.uk

Mental health charity that supports students.

Tommy's

tommys.org
Information and support for people affected by stillbirth,
miscarriage and premature birth.

YoungMinds

0808 802 5544 (parents helpline)
85258 (crisis messenger service, text YM)
youngminds.org.uk
Committed to improving the mental health of babies, children
and young people, including support for parents and carers.

Support for people experiencing suicidal thoughts

Mind's services

- Helplines – information and support by phone, email
  and text.

- Local Minds – provide face-to-face services across England
  and Wales. These might be talking therapies, peer support
  and advocacy.

- Elefriends – our supportive online community for anyone
  experiencing a mental health problem.

Other organisations

Campaign Against Living Miserably (CALM)

0800 58 58 58 (UK helpline)

0808 802 58 58 (London helpline)

thecalmzone.net

Provides listening services, information and support for men at risk of suicide, including a web chat.

Carers UK

0808 808 7777

carersuk.org

Advice and support for people caring for someone else.

Maytree Suicide Respite Centre

020 7263 7070

maytree.org.uk

Offers free respite stays for people in suicidal crisis.

MindOut

mindout.org.uk

Mental health service run by and for LGBTQ+ people.

Papyrus HOPELINEUK

0800 068 41 41

07786 209697 (text)

papyrus-uk.org

Confidential support for under-35s at risk of suicide and others who are concerned about them.

Sane

0300 304 7000

sane.org.uk

Offers emotional support and information for anyone affected by mental health problems.

Samaritans

116 123 (freephone)

jo@samaritans.org

samaritans.org

Open 24/7 for anyone who needs to talk. You can visit some branches in person. They also have a Welsh Language Line on 0300 123 3011 (7pm–11pm every day).

Zero suicide alliance

https://www.zerosuicidealliance.com/training

Stay Alive

prevent-suicide.org.uk

App with help and resources for people who feel suicidal or are supporting someone else.

Survivors of Bereavement by Suicide (SOBS)

0300 111 5065

uk-sobs.org.uk

Emotional and practical support and local groups for anyone bereaved or affected by suicide.

Useful resources for Psychosis:

Bipolar UK

0333 323 3880

bipolaruk.org

Information and support for people affected by bipolar disorder, hypomania and mania.

Hearing Voices Network

hearing-voices.org

Information and support for people who hear voices or have other unshared perceptions, including local support groups.

Mood Diaries

medhelp.org/land/mood-tracker

moodscope.com

moodchart.org

moodpanda.com

Some examples of mood diaries – many more are available. Mind doesn't endorse any particular one.

National Institute for Health and Care Excellence (NICE)

nice.org.uk

Produces guidelines on best practice in healthcare.

National Paranoia Network

nationalparanoianetwork.org

Information and support for people who experience paranoid thoughts.

Rethink Mental Illness

0300 5000 927
rethink.org
Provides support and information for anyone affected by mental health problems, including local support groups.

Samaritans

116 123 (freephone)
jo@samaritans.org
Freepost RSRB-KKBY-CYJK
PO Box 90 90
Stirling FK8 2SA
samaritans.org

Online and phone support for children and young people:

Childline

childline.org.uk

- Children can confidentially call, email, or chat online about any problem big or small

- Freephone helpline: 0800 1111 (24 hour service)

- Sign up for a childline account on the website to message a counsellor anytime without email

The Mix

themix.org.uk

- Provides a confidential helpline, email, webchat and telephone counselling service for young people under 25. Advice and information on support services for young people including counselling.

- Freephone: 0808 808 4994 (daily 13:00-23:00)

Kooth

kooth.com

- Provides free, safe, anonymous online support for young people - counselling, messaging, personal stories. Only available in certain parts of England and Wales.

Relate (for children and young people)

relate.org.uk

- Children and young people's counselling for any young person who's having problems.

- Free Live Chat session with a trained Relate Counsellor

- Phone: 0300 100 1234

Royal College of Psychiatrists – You Can Cope

rcpsych.ac.uk

https://www.rcpsych.ac.uk/mental-health/parents-and-young-people/young-people/u-can-cope!-how-to-cope-when-life-is-difficult-for-young-people

Other organisations and charities specifically for children and young people:

Resources:

Action for Children -

www.actionforchildren.org.uk

Anna Freud National Centre for Children and Families

www.annafreud.org

BACP

www.bacp.co.uk

Barnardo's

www.barnardos.org.uk

Beat

www.beateatingdisorders.org.uk

BYC – British Youth Council

www.byc.org.uk

Carers Trust

carers.org

Centre for Mental Health

www.centreformentalhealth.org.uk

CWMT

charliewaller.org

Family Action

www.family-action.org.uk

Foundation for People with Learning Disabilities

www.learningdisabilities.org.uk

Mental Health Foundation

https://www.mentalhealth.org.uk/

MHFA – Mental Health First Aid England

mhfaengland.org

MindEd

www.minded.org.uk

NSPCC

www.nspcc.org.uk

Place 2 Be

www.place2be.org.uk

RC Psych

www.rcpsych.ac.uk

RCPCH

www.rcpch.ac.uk

Rethink Mental Illness

www.rethink.org

Royal College of Nursing

www.rcn.org.uk

Tavistock Relationships

www.tavistockrelationships.org

The Association for Child and Adolescent Mental Health

www.acamh.org

The British Psychological Society

www.bps.org.uk

The Children's Society

www.childrenssociety.org.uk

The Mix
www.themix.org.uk

Winston's Wish
www.winstonswish.org

Young Minds
youngminds.org.uk

Youth Access
www.youthaccess.org.uk

Further detail on some of the above resources:

Young Minds Crisis Messenger

Provides free, 24/7 text support for young people across the UK experiencing a mental health crisis.

All texts are answered by trained volunteers, with support from experienced clinical supervisors.

Texts are free from EE, O2, Vodafone, 3, Virgin Mobile, BT Mobile, GiffGaff, Tesco Mobile and Telecom Plus.

Texts can be anonymous, but if the volunteer believes you are at immediate risk of harm, they may share your details with people who can provide support.

Text: YM to 85258   Opening times: 24/7

Beat

beateatingdisorders.org.uk

- Offers information and support for anybody affected by eating disorders.

- One-to-one web chat available.

- Enter your postcode in the Help Finder to see what eating disorder support is available in your area.

Information on helpline accessibility and confidentiality available here.

Phone: 0808 801 0677 (helpline for anyone over 18)

Phone: 0808 801 0711 (youth line for anyone under 18)

Phone: 0808 801 0811 (student line)

Email: help@beateatingdisorders.org.uk (for anyone over 18)

Email: fyp@beateatingdisorders.org.uk (for anyone under 18)

Email: studentline@beateatingdisorders.org.uk (for students)

Opening times: 365 days a year - weekdays (9am - 8pm); weekends (4pm - 8pm)

Anorexia and Bulimia Care

anorexiabulimiacare.org.uk

- Offers support to anyone affected by eating disorders.

- Hosts an online community for anybody supporting someone with an eating disorder.

Email: support@anorexiabulimiacare.org.uk (support for individuals with an eating disorder)

Email: familyandfriends@anorexiabulimiacare.org.uk (support for family and friends)

Phone: 03000 11 12 13 (9am - 1pm; 2pm - 5pm, Wednesday - Friday)

Opening times: 9:30am - 5pm, Tuesday - Friday

The Mix

themix.org.uk

- Essential support for anyone under 25 about anything that's troubling them.

- Email support available via their online contact form.

- Free 1-2-1 webchat service available.

- Free short-term counselling service available.

Phone: 0808 808 4994

Opening times: 4pm - 11pm, seven days a week

Youth Access

youthaccess.org.uk

- Provides information about local counselling and advice services for young people aged 12-25.

British Association for Counselling and Psychotherapy (BACP)

- Professional body that sets standards for therapeutic practice, and provides information for therapists, clients of therapy, and the general public. Website includes information about counselling and psychotherapy and how to find the right therapist.

Phone: 01455 883 300 (Mon-Fri 09:00 – 17:00)

Association of Child Psychotherapists

- A register of accredited Child and Adolescent Psychotherapists in the UK. Name search function on website of all who are eligible and available to work in private practice. It aims to uphold high standards in training and practice.

Counselling Directory

- Lists private counsellors and psychotherapists who are registered by a professional body. They also provide information on the different types of talking therapies including family therapy.

British Psychological Society

- Information on how psychologists can help with mental health problems, and how to find a psychologist.

Youth Wellbeing Directory

- Lists of local services for young people's mental health and wellbeing.

Counselling for families - Relate

Support, guidance and counselling services for families and young people. When families are going through a tough time, relate offers support to help everyone settle. Phone: 0300 100 1234 or contact your local Relate Centre.

- Relate (for families)

- Relate (for family life and parenting)

- Relate (parenting teenagers)

- Relate counselling options: Live chatroom, message a counsellor, webcam counselling, telephone counselling

Online and phone support for children and young people:

childline

- Children can confidentially call, email, or chat online about any problem big or small

- Freephone helpline: 0800 1111 (24 hour service)

- Sign up for a childline account on the website to message a counsellor anytime without email

The Mix

- Provides a confidential helpline, email, webchat and telephone counselling service for young people under 25. Advice and information on support services for young people including counselling.

- Freephone: 0808 808 4994 (daily 13:00-23:00)

Kooth

- Provides free, safe, anonymous online support for young people - counselling, messaging, personal stories. Only available in certain parts of England and Wales.

Relate (for children and young people)

- Children and young people's counselling for any young person who's having problems.

- Free Live Chat session with a trained Relate Counsellor

Phone: 0300 100 1234

Self harm

- Mind – call 0300 123 3393 or text 86463 (9am to 6pm on weekdays)

- Harmless – email info@harmless.org.uk

- Self-injury Support (for women and girls)

- CALM (for men of all ages)

- Young Minds Parents Helpline – call 0808 802 5544 (9.30am to 4pm on weekdays)

- National Self Harm Network forums

If you struggle with suicidal thoughts or are supporting someone else, the Staying Safe website provides information on how to make a safety plan. It includes video tutorials and online templates to guide you through the process.

You could also download the free distrACT app. This gives you easy, quick and discreet access to information and advice about self-harm and suicidal thoughts.

Alumina – free online help for people self-harming

www.selfharm.co.uk- free online self-harm support for 14-19s

Other more general mental health first aid resources:

MIND has a page of helpful pointers that may be useful for someone reticent about speaking about a possible mental health issue: seeking help for a mental health problem

You can cope – advice for Young People

rcpsych.ac.uk

https://www.rcpsych.ac.uk/mental-health/parents-and-young-people/young-people/u-can-cope!-how-to-cope-when-life-is-difficult-for-young-people

- Health & Safety Executive (HSE): www.hse.gov.uk

- Skills for Health: www.skillsforhealth.org.uk

- Mind: www.mind.org.uk

- Mental Health Foundation: www.mentalhealth.org.uk

- NICE: www.nice.org.uk/search?q=mental+health

- Samaritans: www.samaritans.org

- Rethink mental illness: www.rethink.org/services-groups/ service-types/advice-and-helplines

- Anxiety UK: www.anxietyuk.org.uk

- Citizen advice: www.citizensadvice.org.uk

- MindEd: www.minded.org.uk

- Mental Health UK: www.mentalhealth-uk.org

- Bipolar UK: www.bipolaruk.org.uk

- Calm: www.thecalmzone.net

- Mens Health Forum: www.menshealthforum.org.uk

- No Panic: www.nopanic.org.uk

- OCD Action: www.ocdaction.org.uk

- OCD UK: www.ocduk.org

- Papyrus: www.papyrus-uk.org

- SANE: www.sane.org.uk/support

- Young Minds: www.youngminds.org.uk

- NSPCC: www.nspcc.org.uk

- Refuge: www.refuge.org.uk

- Alcoholics Anonymous: www.alcoholics-anonymous.org.uk

- Gamblers Anonymous: www.gamblersanonymous.org.uk

- Narcotics Anonymous: www.ukna.org

- Alzheimer's Society: www.alzheimers.org.uk

- Cruse Bereavement Care: www.cruse.org.uk

- Rape Crisis: www.rapecrisis.org.uk

- Victim Support: www.victimsupport.org

- Beat: www.b-eat.co.uk

- Mencap: www.mencap.org.uk

- Family Lives: www.familylives.org.uk

- Relate: www.relate.org.uk

Mental health conditions, work and the workplace

The Stevenson Farmer 'Thriving at Work' review

In 2017, the government commissioned Lord Stevenson and Paul Farmer (Chief Executive of Mind) to independently review how employers can better support individuals with mental health conditions in the workplace.

The resulting HSE's Management Standards approach to tackling work-related stress established a framework to help employers improve their approach to mental health in the workplace and stress in particular and consequently reduce the incidence and negative impact of mental ill health.

The Management Standards approach creates a framework to help employers manage work-related stress.

Example stress policy (HSE)

https://www.hse.gov.uk/stress/mental-health.htm

The HSE Stress Workbook

https://www.hse.gov.uk/pubns/wbk01.pdf

References:

McManus, S., Meltzer, H., Brugha, T. S., Bebbington, P. E., & Jenkins, R. (2009). Adult psychiatric morbidity in England, 2007: results of a household survey.

McManus S, Bebbington P, Jenkins R, Brugha T. (eds.) (2016). Mental health and wellbeing in England: Adult psychiatric morbidity survey 2014.

Samaritans (2019), Samaritans Suicide Statistics Report.

WHO (2003). Caring for children and adolescents with mental disorders: Setting WHO directions. [online] Geneva: World Health Organization. Available at: http://www.who.int/mental_health/media/en/785.pdf [Accessed 14 Sep. 2015].

https://digital.nhs.uk/news-and-events/news/survey-conducted-in-july-2020-shows-one-in-six-children-having-a-probable-mental-disorder

Kessler RC, Berglund P, Demler O, Jin R, Merikangas KR, Walters EE. (2005). Lifetime Prevalence and Age-of-Onset Distributions of DSM-IV Disorders in the National Comorbidity Survey Replication. Archives of General Psychiatry, 62 (6) pp. 593-602. doi:10.1001/archpsyc.62.6.593.

Green,H., Mcginnity, A., Meltzer, Ford, T., Goodman,R. 2005 Mental Health of Children and Young People in Great Britain: 2004. Office for National Statistics.

Children's Society (2008) The Good Childhood Inquiry: health research evidence. London: Children's Society.

Printed in Great Britain
by Amazon